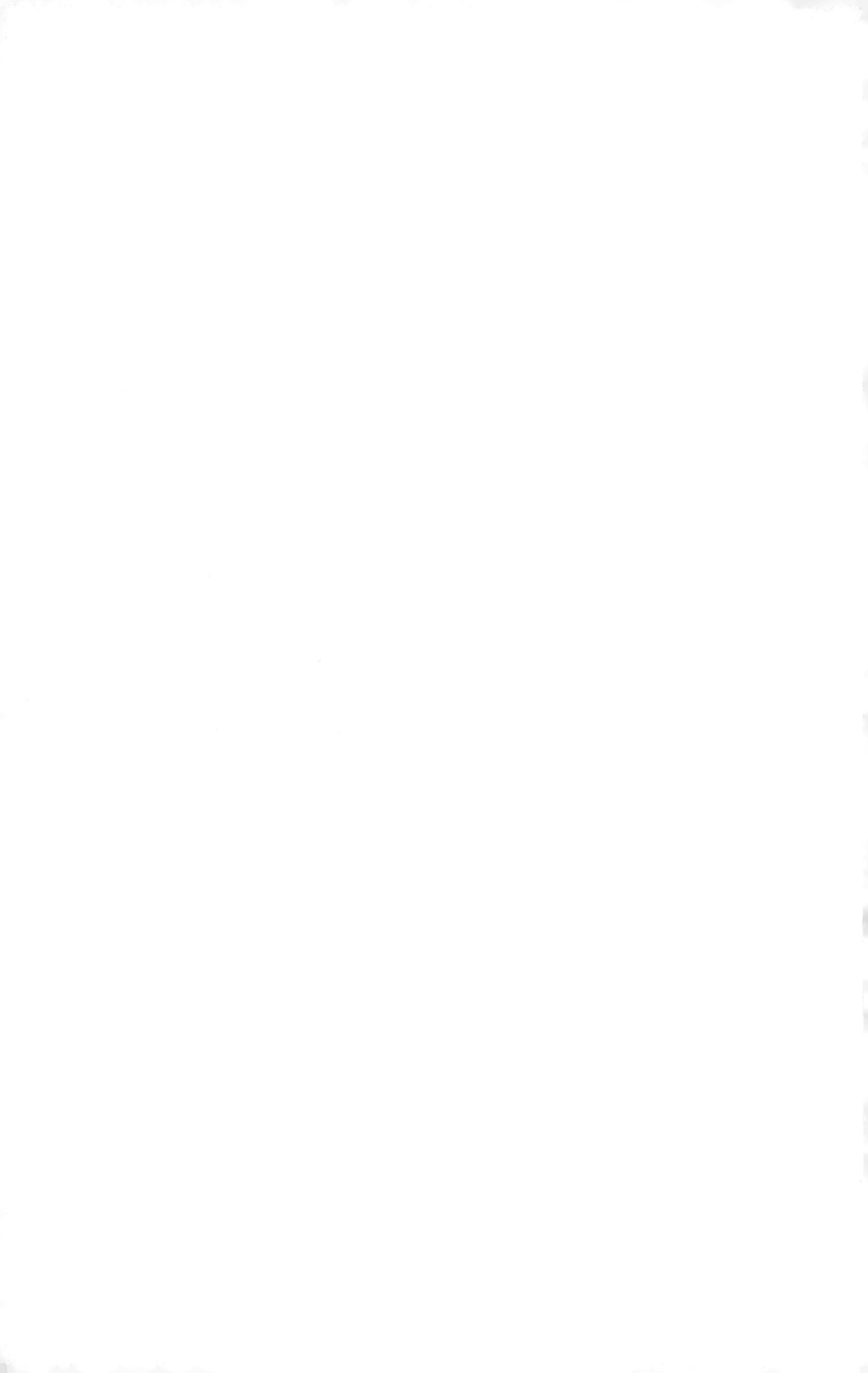

You Can Heal
NATURALLY

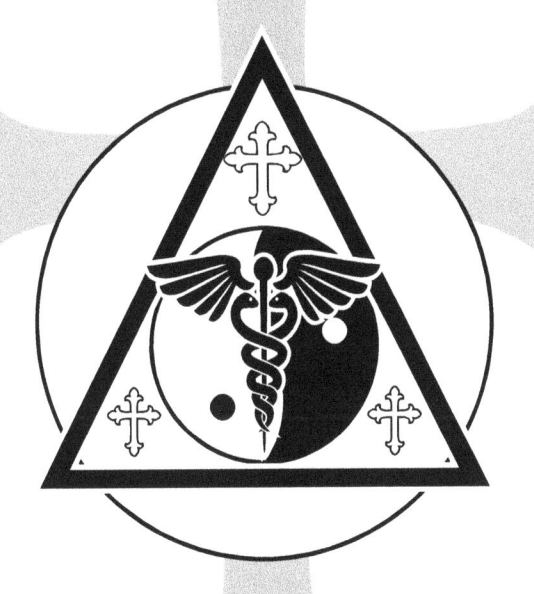

Learn the Art and Science of Muscle Testing

Dr. Jerry Weber, ND

BALBOA.PRESS
A DIVISION OF HAY HOUSE

Copyright © 2021 Dr. Jerry Weber, ND.

All rights reserved. No part of this book may be used or reproduced by any means, graphic, electronic, or mechanical, including photocopying, recording, taping or by any information storage retrieval system without the written permission of the author except in the case of brief quotations embodied in critical articles and reviews.

Balboa Press books may be ordered through booksellers or by contacting:

Balboa Press
A Division of Hay House
1663 Liberty Drive
Bloomington, IN 47403
www.balboapress.com
844-682-1282

Because of the dynamic nature of the Internet, any web addresses or links contained in this book may have changed since publication and may no longer be valid. The views expressed in this work are solely those of the author and do not necessarily reflect the views of the publisher, and the publisher hereby disclaims any responsibility for them.

The author of this book does not dispense medical advice or prescribe the use of any technique as a form of treatment for physical, emotional, or medical problems without the advice of a physician, either directly or indirectly. The intent of the author is only to offer information of a general nature to help you in your quest for emotional and spiritual well-being. In the event you use any of the information in this book for yourself, which is your constitutional right, the author and the publisher assume no responsibility for your actions.

Any people depicted in stock imagery provided by Getty Images are models, and such images are being used for illustrative purposes only.
Certain stock imagery © Getty Images.

Print information available on the last page.

ISBN: 978-1-9822-6690-5 (sc)
ISBN: 978-1-9822-6696-7 (hc)
ISBN: 978-1-9822-6691-2 (e)

Library of Congress Control Number: 2021907232

Balboa Press rev. date: 07/08/2021

CONTENTS

Acknowledgements.. vii
Foreword... ix
Introduction... xv

LEVEL 1: BEGINNER

Chapter 1   This Book Could Save Your Health 1
Chapter 2   What Will You Do When You Get Sick? 7
Chapter 3   Everything Is Energy – Including You 13
Chapter 4   The Art and Science of Muscle Testing........... 23

LEVEL 2: INTERMEDIATE

Chapter 5   The Body Balance Healing System 51
Chapter 6   The Circulatory System – The Deliverer 59
Chapter 7   The Digestive System – the Food Processor ... 67
Chapter 8   The Intestinal System – You Food Transporter ... 83
Chapter 9   The Glandular (Endocrine) System –
            Your Hormone Supplier 95
Chapter 10 Immune/Lymphatic System – The Protector... 105
Chapter 11 The Nervous System – Your Information Carrier...113
Chapter 12 The Respiratory System – Your Oxygen Deliverer ... 125
Chapter 13 The Reproductive System – The Giver of Life ...131
Chapter 14 The Structural System – The Foundation 141
Chapter 15 The Urinary System – Your Balancer 149
Chapter 16 The Cause of Disease..................................... 153

LEVEL 3: ADVANCED

Chapter 17 Emotional Release Therapy............................163
Chapter 18 It's All About Frequency – The Secret 169

Appendix 177

ACKNOWLEDGEMENTS

I first would like to thank God for giving me the inspiration, and ability to write this book.

I would like to thank Ann - my wife, and co-partner in life. She is the inspiration of my life. I would never be doing what I am honored to do without her support, understanding and sacrifice.

I would like to thank my two editors, Virginia Berry and Susan Crisafulli. They both were instrumental in bringing these words to print in the best form possible.

I would like to thank Carol Bosmeny for constructing all the wonderful charts. She was able to take my craziness of numbers and topics and organize them into a perfect learning tool.

I would like to thank Dr. Cliff Fetters for taking time away from his family, and business, to write the forward for this book. I also want to thank him for believing in me, and allowing me to work beside him. It is an honor and blessing.

I would like to thank our son, Dr. Michael Weber, for his input, and support building the Body Balance Healing System over the last ten years.

I would like to thank Cassidy Waters, our social media guru, for helping me get our message to the world.

I would like to thank the "models" in the book – Antionette, April, Yvonne, and Rocky

I would like to thank Harry O for his expertise, knowledge, testimony, and advice.

I would like to thank Bud Tarentto for his testimony, support and friendship

I would like to thank all of my teachers, patients, fellow practitioners, and students for joining me on this journey of natural health. Thank you for trusting me, and allowing me to be your guide. God bless all of you.

FOREWORD

I was trained in traditional medicine with a MD degree from Indiana University followed by three-year residency program in family medicine. It took me less than one year in private practice to realize that using prescription drugs to mask the symptoms of chronic diseases was not the solution. After being acquainted with holistic and functional medicine, I became enthralled with discovering a natural solution for all ailments. My mission is to usher holistic medicine into mainstream healthcare. It is agonizing to observe so many Americans living in pain from chronic illnesses when I know they can benefit greatly from holistic treatment.

In 2010, I had been practicing holistic/functional medicine for over 20 years. With so much experience, I was confident enough to tell my patients that I could help at least 95% of them achieve optimal wellness. I did not pay attention until after my third patient reminded me that she was one of my five percenters I could not help. She therefore sought help elsewhere and she was healed. This was the third time a patient told me that they had consulted with a naturopathic doctor named Jerry Weber.

She explained in detail how this naturopath went through every organ system and measured the exact function of each body system. He then tested all the possible pathogens that could be harming each system. She was told that her decade old postoperative paralyzed hemidiaphragm was due to a viral infection rather than from an accidental slip of a surgeon's knife. He treated her only with natural herbs and supplements based upon muscle testing. I was quite skeptical. It sounded too easy. I had known her for a very long time, and I knew she was a credible witness. Upon her return to me, she was no longer having respiratory difficulties. I was shocked to see both normal pulmonary function tests and a chest x-ray that revealed the hemidiaphragm had returned to a normal position. Ten years later, she is still doing well.

Two additional patients also had a precise diagnosis and successful treatment. He still sounded too good to be true. I determined that the best way to check out this talent was to become a patient myself. In less than a 60-minute appointment, he was able to come up with my complete assessment.

I am a rare physician who practices what he preaches, and I can say that his complete assessment was consistent with the results of thousands of dollars' worth of labs and specialized testing. After our second visit, I was convinced that Jerry and I had to work together. Fortunately, I was able make him an offer he could not refuse.

This was one of the best decisions of my medical career. The Body Balance Healing System method of muscle testing has allowed me to be much more precise and efficient in my evaluation and treatment process. Now my patients rarely have any side effects or bad reactions to protocols. The charting system makes it easy to consider a great number of possible problems that could potentially be the root cause of disease. This gift often guides me in the right direction and ultimately to a conclusion thus saving my patients thousands of dollars' worth of unnecessary laboratory test and radiation exposure from x-rays. The ability to test remotely saves countless hours for myself and my patients.

New healthcare providers are often concerned about negative perception from their patients with the use of muscle testing. I simply quote Dr. Weber, "results are what matters." We are simply making decisions based upon the energy from another diagnostic tool. Most medical doctors that practice functional medicine at the highest level are master muscle testers. Where does energy come from and how can we tap into it? Most people believe in a higher power whether they call it God, quantum physics, universal knowledge, the Holy Spirit, etc. My belief is in the Holy Spirit and we are simply asking God for the truth. The bottom line is that Dr. Weber's system has allowed me to give patients a more precise and accurate treatment plan allowing 99% the potential to achieve optimal wellness.

We currently have amazing technology in the field of blood chemistries, detecting infectious diseases and high-resolution imaging. Most diagnostic testing is expensive and radiation from imaging can be harmful. Moreover, no test is absolute. The beauty of muscle testing is that it's free and without radiation exposure. The mastery is in the questions you ask, the interpretations that you make and the ideal plan from the discovery.

Muscle testing is not just for healthcare providers. Many of my employees and patients have taken a course provided by Dr. Weber. Once proficient, one can incorporate muscle testing in all realms of daily living. I do not buy nor consume food or drinks without muscle testing. I muscle test all skin and hair products for potential toxins. I muscle test environments for mold toxins as well as toxic electromagnetic fields. I have found that after many years of muscle testing, I have greatly improved my natural intuition. Sometimes you just know in your mind what is true. I can better pick up on other people's energy and emotions which allows me to help others. The wonderful technology from the modern world can sometimes make life confusing and overwhelming. Dr. Weber's methods empower individuals to take more control of their health by tapping into universal knowledge and understanding. I have personally derived much peace in knowing that I am on the right path.

The added benefit of working with Dr. Weber is to be in the presence of a man is so compassionate about helping others. He is constantly reading books from every genre of holistic healing. His positive energy and love for others has made him the #1 cheerleader for our entire office. I have never seen him in a bad mood. His positive energy is contagious to all that have the pleasure to be around him. His door is always open for me and my staff to help solve any life problem.

—**Dr. Cliff Fetters**, M.D.

"When health is absent wisdom cannot reveal itself, art cannot manifest, strength cannot fight, wealth becomes useless and intelligence cannot be applied,"

                        Herophilus (Greek physician)

INTRODUCTION

You Can Heal – Naturally has been written to help you empower yourself to take control of your health and the health of your loved ones. Its purpose is to give you the freedom of choice about your health care. You no longer have to be forced into the prevailing and failing "healthcare" system. You now have a choice of the medical approach, taking a more natural path or using both. It is your choice. You will no longer be pushed into the medical system by necessity. You do have another option – a natural approach. That is power!

With this information you learn how to get answers to your health concerns that the medical community has not been able to provide. This book is different. It doesn't discuss diet or what herbs might possibly work. Instead, it provides a step-by-step proven system, which I have been using for years and have helped thousands of people improve their health. *You Can Heal - Naturally* gives you the tools and information to find the answers about your health you have been praying for. All you have to do is have the faith to believe, step out of your comfort zone, try something new and put this program into your life. Your body will love you for it.

Your health is the most important asset you possess. Your body is the temple that God has created. It is your responsibility and challenge to keep this temple as strong and vital as humanly possible. You no longer have to trust your health to a system that looks at you as an insurance number more than a real person. In your hands you have the vehicle to a healthier future *if* you choose to use it. You are now in the driver's seat. It is like any information. It is only as good as the effort you put in to it. Take the time and effort to read, learn and apply this system. It will be well worth the investment. Invest in yourself, it always pays the highest interest.

No one knows your body better than you do. No one understands how you feel. No one else has their life on the line when your health is concerned. It is *your* life and *your* health. Do something about it. Learn how to keep yourself and your loved ones healthier - not by a new diet or pill, but rather by using easy muscle testing techniques, and a proven healthcare system. That is exactly what You Can Heal – Naturally can do.

"Unless we put medical freedom into the Constitution the time will come when medicine will organize into an undercover dictatorship. To restrict the art of healing to one class of men and deny equal to others will constitute the Bastille of medical science. All such laws are un-American and despotic and have no place in a republic. The Constitution of the republic should make special privilege for medical freedom as well as religion freedom."

Dr. Benjamin Rush, MD.
(signer of the Declaration of Independence and physician to George Washington)

The time has come…

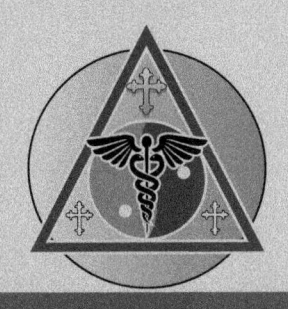

LEVEL 1

BEGINNER

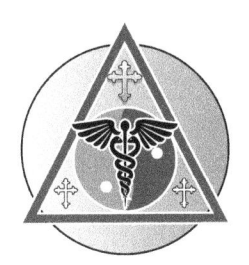

CHAPTER ONE

This Book Could Save Your Health

Let's face it - America is sick! We are no longer "the land of the free and home of the brave." We now are "the land of the addicted and home of the pharmaceutical cartels." The truth is a majority of Americans are using prescription medications.

A study from Mayo Clinic states 20% of Americans take at least five pharmaceutical drugs. (Zhong et al 2013). The same study also shows that 50% of Americans take at least two medications, and 70% are using at least one prescription.

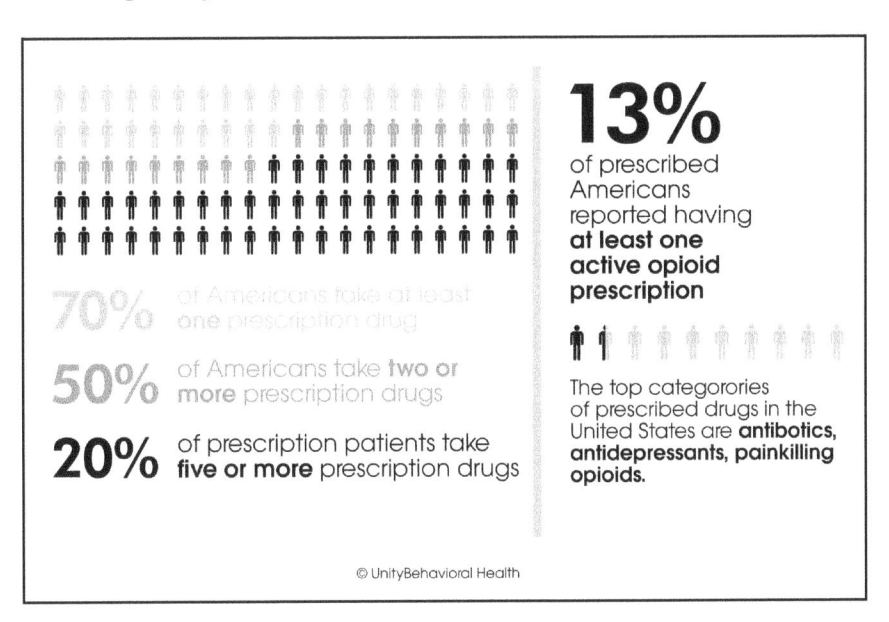

70% of Americans take at least one prescription drug

50% of Americans take **two or more** prescription drugs

20% of prescription patients take **five or more** prescription drugs

13% of prescribed Americans reported having **at least one active opioid prescription**

The top categorories of prescribed drugs in the United States are **antibotics, antidepressants, painkilling opioids.**

© UnityBehavioral Health

Our nation is not strong. A country cannot be strong and self-reliant when the majority of its citizens are required to use drugs to function for the day. Parents tell their kids, "stay away from drugs," as they take their

YOU CAN HEAL NATURALLY • 1

daily prescribed dosage. A person is not free when hooked on a daily drug to sustain life – even when it is prescribed. Yes, these people are living but not getting healthier.

I understand that some people will not agree, and argue they absolutely need their medications. They are right. These people will be using the same drugs, and more, for the rest of their lives. Because of fear, lack of desire, or disbelief, they refuse to regain their health, and instead rely on these "crutches" to cope. They do not believe they can heal. Some people are in such severe imbalance, and disease, they must use the medications. Thank God for these medications to help people stay alive, and out of pain. But let's make it perfectly clear. These types of drugs will never make you healthier. For a truly healthy life you must choose a more natural route.

I remember attending a demonstration where a person was speaking about using intuition. A person asked the question, "do pharmaceutical medications affect your intuitive abilities?" The speaker answered 'no." I was shocked that he said that, and I blurted out. "That's not true," As soon as the words escaped my mouth, I was bombarded by a lady sitting next to me, who said she couldn't possibly go off her thyroid or her blood pressure medicine. To her surprise, I agreed with her, and then added, "all I said, was that I don't believe synthetic medications don't affect the bodies intuitive abilities." I absolutely believe that all synthetic substances, including medications, affect the body in a negative manner.

How could anybody believe that pharmaceutical medications *don't* affect the body in a negative way? They absolutely do. They numb the senses, block receptors, and affect every function in the body. If you don't believe me, watch the television ads. Listen to the voice in the background, talking rapidly telling you about all the "side effects" of this "wonderful drug". Watch the happy couple, frolicking through the field of sunflowers, having the time of their life, as though they were thirty something again. It looks good – maybe *too* good.

I absolutely believe in medical treatment, pharmaceutical medications, and even surgery when it is absolutely necessary. The truth is that these medical options have saved millions of lives. Thank God for medicine. But, it doesn't treat the "root cause" of the health concern. Prescription medicine forces you into a lifetime of pharmaceutical dependence, with medications getting more expensive. Medication makes you a victim. You think "there's nothing I can do except take this medication, as my doctor ordered."

The fact is: our society is getting sicker, more obese, stressed and depressed. Deaths from prescription drugs and medical treatment rank as the third largest killer, just behind cancer and heart disease, causing over 100,000 deaths every year in the U.S. Suicide rates are climbing. More murders are happening on our streets. Our society is an addicted race of over-used, over-prescribed, harmful, pharmaceutical medications that do not address the "root cause."

I believe my mother was killed by the daily use of excessive, prescribed medications, from her medical doctor. She was taking eight different medications, including Coumadin– the blood thinning drug, which includes Warfarin - rat poison. The sad fact is there are millions of people being prescribed poisons in the name of "health care."

Mom had to go every week to her doctor to get her blood checked, to make sure it was not too thin. Over the Christmas holidays, my wife fixed a beautiful green salad and took it to my mother. She absolutely loved it – until she went in to see her doctor the next week. After doing an exam, the doctor was alarmed, and asked her what she had changed. She told the medical professional how Ann had fixed her a green salad, and she had eaten it all. The doctor exploded, "You can't eat greens. They will make your blood too thin!" Which is exactly what the blood test proved.

My mother reported to me about her doctor telling her she couldn't eat any more greens because they made her blood too thin. I had to ask the obvious question. "Then why not eat the greens every day, and not take the Coumadin?" Her answer motivated me to write this book. She answered, with total sincerity, "My doctor told me that I can't stop the medication. If I do, it might kill me." I believe that being *on* the medication killed her.

My father-in-law, Bill, who had previously suffered a stroke, was also on many medications. Because of a problem between VA and the insurance company, one of his medications was switched to a cheaper generic substitute. After taking the very first of his new medication before going to bed, he died in his sleep.

At six months old, our daughter, Leslie, suffered 105 fever, and convulsions immediately after her first round of baby vaccinations. Taking her back to the doctor as recommended, the pediatrician prescribed an epileptic narcotic, that she would be on for nine years! He didn't even do any testing, assuming it *might* be epilepsy, and "prescribing" a harmful drug for a baby to take for nine years! At that point, my wife and I both refused to succumb to such an outrageous proposition, and said. "no," took our baby, and left the office, never to return.

Within three days, a lady from Child Protective Services was knocking on our door. We had been reported to the agency, accused as "unfit parents." Because we would not blindly go along with this "professional's" opinion, we instantly became "bad parents." And all we were doing was trying to protect our baby. I explained to the lady we were not trying to harm our child, but felt there was a better answer – a more natural approach for this problem. I also added, that we didn't believe without further testing, that our child could be properly diagnosed with epilepsy – which the doctor used as the reason for prescribing such a harmful drug for the most formative years. We promised her we would find an answer, and we did. Because of this experience, Ann and I started our lifetime journey of natural health and healing.

Today, because of our decision, Leslie is a healthy, happy, forty-year old with a loving husband of fifteen years and five "fur babies." But what if we had listened, and followed the doctor's orders?

Years later I was shown the other scenario. I met a lady, about Leslie's age. She was with her mother, and it was obvious that the daughter had mental disabilities. As we talked, I heard a story that sounded like "déjà vu." Her mother told me that after her daughter's first baby shots she had a fever, and convulsions. The doctor prescribed the exact same medication he wanted to put Leslie on. Because of that narcotic drug, this young lady was mentally crippled for the rest of her life. Her mother cried, "We didn't know any better. We did what we thought was right. We trusted the doctor."

These are just some of the personal stories that motivated me to write You Can Heal – Naturally. If this book helps even one person save their health, it is a success. I believe it can give you the information you need so you and your family never have to experience these types of situations. This book gives you a proven system you can use to take more control of your health, and have the information to make the best choice possible when you do get sick.

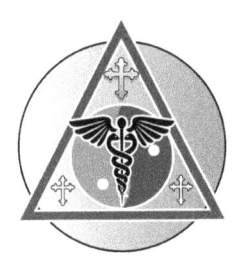

CHAPTER TWO

What Will You Do When You Get Sick?

Health is wealth. Nobody can argue that fact. Most of us are blessed and born healthy. We grow up with excess energy and drive and feel that we are invincible until some type of health crisis happens. We take our health for granted, until it disappears. If you lose your health you lose everything. You sacrifice the ability to enjoy the life you've dreamed about and deserve. It creates emotional and financial stress which causes a downward spiral of frustration, pain and disease. Disease stops you from living the life that God has planned for you.

All of us will get sick during our lifetime. Whether it is a minor cough or a major life-threatening disease you will face a time when you will have to make a decision on what you are going to do to get well. The obvious choice for the majority of Americans is to schedule an appointment with their family MD, emergency room or urgent care.

But, is this always the best choice to choose for optimum health? I don't think so.

The choice you make during this health crisis could negatively affect your health for the rest of your life. I have talked to many patients who made choices about their health that they now wish they had not made. If only they had known.

In all due respect to all the hardworking, dedicated medical professionals the answer is NO. The answer might shock you and go against your programmed beliefs. Allow me to explain why this thinking might not be the best approach for optimal health for you or your family.

Our modern medical healthcare system in the United States, which most Americans rely on, is not designed to be a "health care system." It actually is a "sick care system" that focuses on eradicating the germ or disease once you get it. We have the best "sick care system" in the world. Our emergency medical care is outstanding and saves many lives every day. These professionals are doing the job they were trained to do and doing a great job of it. But, none of these wonderful, needed services qualify as a "health care service."

Don't get me wrong. If I have a medical emergency, rush me to the best medical doctor that money can buy (and it takes a lot). But, for all other minor aches and pains our doctors don't have any reasonable answers. For medical emergencies, pharma drugs and surgery are the answer to save a person's life. But these two options cannot possibly heal the body. Yes, these medications can kill the pain – for a while. But they never address the "root cause" of why the body is in pain. That is what The Body Balance Healing System can do for you.

If you truly desire vibrant health you must learn about natural health. You must learn how to "read" the body's cry for help. It's not about a miracle product. It is about a simple system of health care that you can learn and use in the privacy of your home. This approach might not be as easy as just following the doctor's orders. It will cost you more because insurance doesn't pay for most natural health products. But if you don't make the investment and decide to follow the well-worn path of society your future could look bleak.

When a person continues using medications long term it is not a pretty picture. All the "side effects" over time take a toll on the body, and become "direct effects." Take a few minutes and visit a local nursing home, or watch people. How are they walking? Ask them how they feel. Do they have energy? Are they healthy? Do you want to be like them in the near future? I believe you will see people who are in pain, obese, exhausted, unhappy, limping, and exhibiting the signs of a body, and brain that is deteriorating. Most of these suffering souls are on medications. Something isn't working. If you want the same results, follow their lead down the well-worn, drug lined path. It is simple to do, and insurance will pay for most of it, but... if you want to live a healthy life at any age, natural health is the only choice.

More adults are on pharmaceutical drugs than ever before in the history of our country. More children are being forced on medications before they are out of elementary school. They quickly create a habit of needing their fix whether it is legal or illegal drugs. We are experiencing the worst epidemic of deaths from prescribed medications and illegal over doses and it keeps increasing every year. More families are being broken apart because of addicted drug use. Every family is being negatively affected in some way. Something is not working.

Don't be like these people. Don't follow the crowd down the path of despair and disease. Get more informed. Learn how to help your body stay healthier. You cannot count on someone else to keep you healthy. It is your responsibility to do that. Doctors are there to help you in a crisis. Your goal should be not to let your body get so far out of balance that your body digresses to disease. Disease is dis-ease. Dis-ease is the lack of ease or excess stress in the body.

There are many minor symptoms caused by different facets of stress that your body is trying to get you to pay attention before the "big one" attacks you. By knowing how to muscle test you will be able to correct these small problems before they turn into those big, scary ones. Don't let this happen to you.

If you don't know how to muscle test, you will go through all the frustration, time, and expense, of riding the medical merry-go-round. Instead, by learning these simple muscle testing skills and knowledge of this system, you will be able to find the root cause of any symptom, and correct it with a natural remedy. Choosing this approach, you will not have any side effects. Which one makes the most sense to you?

America Needs an Attitude Adjustment

To get better control of your health you have to change your belief system about the current medical profession, the FDA and the pharmaceutical cartel. Any belief you now have that does not empower you to take better care of yourself and family, needs to be changed. Any belief that makes you feel victimized must be changed to truly get healthy. To change your beliefs, you must change your thinking. To get a new perspective about your health, you will need more knowledge. You also need a proven method of using this specialized knowledge.

The goal and purpose of <u>You Can Heal – Naturally</u> is to empower you to take more control of your health. This is not a book to teach you about how to eat, exercise, or the latest fad diet. Rather, it will share with you a proven, duplicable system of natural health care that you can learn, and use to keep yourself and your loved ones healthier.

I have helped thousands of patients resolve their health concerns using The Body Balance Healing System. I know it can help you, if you give it a chance. I hope and pray you are ready, willing and able to take this information, and use it to stay as healthy as possible. A true way of healing is in your hands. This information has been given to me by the Holy Spirit to share with the world. You deserve to be healthy. <u>You Can Heal - Naturally</u> will start you on your journey of true healing. Enjoy the ride.

There Is an Answer

Do you really believe that your body can heal naturally? Ask yourself this important question, and then feel your body. Be aware of any negative impulses, thoughts, or reactions. If you experience any hesitation, please read these next examples of how well the body can heal naturally. If you already muscle test, state;

"I believe that my body can heal naturally."

Then muscle test yourself to make sure you believe it. If the muscle test result is weak, that suggests that you consciously and/or subconsciously don't believe it can happen. You have to believe in your heart, with all your soul, you can heal – not just say it. If there is any doubt it will sabotage the healing.

Your body has an innate ability to heal naturally. A good example is when I cut my thumb severely. Most people would have rushed to the emergency room, or urgent care, and received stitches, but not me. I did nothing but clean it, poured colloidal silver into the cut, applied Aloe Vera on the cut, put the skin back in place, wrapped a bandage around it, and thanked God for the healing. I repeated that same steps daily until it was healed.

Today a person couldn't tell what thumb I tried to cut off. It healed back perfectly, with not too much interference. My wife dropped boiling water on herself twice, which resulted in huge blisters and pain. Both times we used the same protocol, and in both situations, the body healed naturally. There is very little evidence of these terrible accidents even happening. Yes, the body wants to heal, and it can do it naturally, which is the way that God intended for the body to function. All you have to know is what to do to help it heal.

We have never been taught how to heal our bodies. We were always programmed to rely on the "smart" doctors. They were the ones that went to school. The truth is, doctors don't heal. Medications don't heal. Herbs don't heal. God heals. Our job is to assist the body in healing, by providing positive, higher conscious thoughts, supplying correct nutrients, removing toxins, and letting the body's magical powers perform a miracle.

When your body is experiencing a symptom, you need to know exactly what to do. This is the reason you go to the doctor, in the first place – you don't know what is wrong, or what to do. That is what <u>*You Can Heal – Naturally*</u> will teach you. This book answers many of the questions you have been asking, but never have been answered. This knowledge will help you take more control of your daily health concerns. By learning the techniques of muscle testing, combined with a systematic blueprint to find the root cause of your health problem, you are on your way to a vibrant and healthier life. Take responsibility for your health. Don't blame anybody, or anything, for your poor health issues.

Understand that to get well it is all up to you. As the old saying goes,

"if it's going to be, it's up to me." That is the truth. Empower yourself with this knowledge, and then apply that knowledge by taking action.

Action produces results, and that is how you get healthier. You must take an active role in your healing. Don't be just a patient, who goes to the doctor as a helpless victim, expecting the doctor to have the magic bullet to heal your pain. You must become a student of health. Learn all you can to keep your body as healthy for as many years as possible. I have a saying; "I have no patience for patients, but I have all the time in the world for a student, who wants to learn how to keep their body healthy." If you want to become a student, just keep reading, and enter the world of natural health and muscle testing.

The first step as a student, of the healing arts, is understanding the concept of energy. I still remember reading my first book about energy. I never realized that little, yellow, book entitled Energy, would start me on a lifetime of learning about this invisible force.

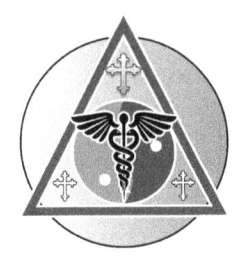

CHAPTER THREE

Everything Is Energy – Including You

"If you want to find the secrets of the Universe (or body), think in terms of energy, frequency, and vibration."
                                                        Nikola Tesla

"Let there be _light_." This scripture from Genesis says it all. <u>Light</u> is <u>energy</u>, and one of the highest frequencies in the Universe. "Let there be _energy_." Why? Because <u>energy</u> is <u>life</u>. "Let there be _life_." Without <u>energy</u> there is no <u>life</u>. When life force (energy of the body) is abundant, this energy is flowing through the body perfectly. The physical signs of this condition is vitality, enthusiasm, joy and good health. This is how God designed us to live – abundant, happy and healthy.

Understanding the concept of energy, and how it relates to keeping the body healthy is crucial. Yet, some fundamental Christians hear the word "energy" and believe it is connected to New Age. Energy is everywhere, and everything. Energy is not just New Age. It is everything in every religion. Being scared of such an important word to understand, is a perfect example of negative programming by religious sects.

When life force energy is blocked, and not flowing through the body properly, the body will react to the stress, and express physical symptoms, such as fatigue, pain, insomnia, headaches and the list goes on, and on. Every symptom you experience, no matter how small it is, the body is trying to communicate to you its need for help. The great news is that your body never lies. It can't lie. All the body is always doing is trying to return to its natural balance of homeostasis.

The answer to this call for help by many people, is to "kill the messenger," with some type of fast acting pain killer. Sometimes this step is necessary, but it is not fixing the problem – only masking it. All prescription drugs either block receptors, slow bodily function down or speed it up. Prescription drugs can't, and never will, truly heal the "root cause" of any health problem.

Why can't prescription medications heal the body? The answer goes back to understanding energy. All prescriptions drugs are man-made, not natural. This defines synthetic. To receive a protective patent on a new drug, there must be a unique factor in that product. Because pure natural nutrients cannot be patented, the pharmaceutical companies chemically change the molecular level so it is "exclusive" to their brand. When the molecular level changes, the frequency or "finger print" of that substance changes. No matter how small, or how good the minor change is reproduced, the cell is smarter. It knows and reacts with a "side-effect", which is actually a direct effect of your body saying "I don't like this. It's not like me." It is very rare when the body reacts to natural supplements. If a person does react to natural supplements or food, it is usually an imbalance in the person's body.

For the body to heal, it must be given 100% natural, organic, herbal supplements, and foods. Supplements, and foods that vibrate at the same frequency as the body should be used. Through muscle testing if the food or supplement makes the muscle strong it is good for the body. The Law of Attraction states that "like attracts like." It is literally impossible to force a foreign, synthetic vibration to become an organic, wholistic vibration that heals the body.

This muscle testing program is the perfect tool for you to use to match your body with the supplements, and foods that work the best for you. We are all individuals, with different needs. What is great for one person, might be terrible for another. Muscle testing is the best technique to confirm what is best for you. How does muscle testing work? It tests the energy flow of your body.

Your goal should be to learn muscle testing, and start applying it in your life. With practice, you will be able to fight off colds, and minor health issues, instead of running to the doctor, and getting an antibiotic. Every time you use natural health, instead of medications, you increase your life force energy.

If you are sick, fatigued or in pain, your life force is blocked, and not flowing properly. How do I know that? Because if the energy (life force) was flowing perfectly, you would feel great. That's how easy it is to get healthier. All you have to do is find the blockages of energy in your body, and correct the imbalance naturally. Once that is accomplished the tissue will regain vital optimum life force, be at the perfect frequency, and reflect optimum health. The goal of natural healing is to obtain optimum functioning in all tissue of every system.

Muscle testing is the best "diagnostic tool" to locate blocked energy flow. The medical professionals are not trained to examine the "micro" level, such as repressed emotions, meridians, tissue or cell level. A competent, knowledgeable, muscle tester can evaluate all these areas, that are "hidden" from the medical eyes. When you learn this program, you will be able to keep yourself, and your family, healthier for the rest of your life.

All energy issues start in the invisible world, and that is why the medical field does not understand. Their left brain, logical nature, will not believe it is truth until it is proven scientifically, to their satisfaction. This energy is called "subtle" energy. This "undetectable" energy cannot be measured by conventional medical equipment. One of the best methods of measuring this invisible energy is muscle testing.

All disease starts in this subtle energy field. EMF disturbance such as radio, or cell phone frequencies, that we can't see, are affecting us every day, decreasing our life force (energy). Wrong foods, negative emotions, excessive stress, chemical imbalances, and toxins from our environment, are all negatively affecting our subtle energy bodies. When life force decreases the physical body slowly begins a downward slide toward disease. When your subtle body's life force increases with the correct thoughts, food, emotions and environment, the body starts a healing process. How do you know which way you are moving – toward health or disease?

How do you feel? That's how you tell which way your health is going. If you have enough energy to do what you want to do, you're doing good. But, what if you just don't have the get-up-and-go you use to have? Lack of energy, not motivated, low libido, unhappy, or sick, are sure signs your energy is not flowing properly.

One of the tools to detect these energy imbalances, is accurate, muscle testing. If you are suffering from any signs of lack of energy, this program is perfect for you.

Now is the time to correct these problems. They're not going to correct themselves. Until the root cause of the imbalance is found, and corrected, the problem will not only persist, but get worse.

Once you learn the fundamentals of muscle testing you will be able to test your own energy. You'll be able to find weakness of energy in your body, with this simple program. Before you start testing, and to make your testing more accurate, understand that all health problems are not always caused by a physical reason. The "root cause" can be in any of the Four Levels of Healing. And only muscle testing can decipher in what layer the primary or secondary cause is located.

The Four Levels of Healing

To understand true healing, you need to be aware of not only what you can see, but also, what you can't see. When it is a physical problem it is obvious. But, what if it isn't obvious? What if it isn't physical? If it isn't physical, what could it be? These are all questions for a student of natural health to ponder, and muscle testing can answer.

There are another three levels of healing besides the physical realm. They are the emotional, mental, and spiritual levels. Each of these areas intertwine with each other. Let's explore each level to understand the importance of these other levels of healing.

The Four Levels of HEALING

100% Source
GOD

(Belief) Spiritual (Lack of Belief)
(Positive) Mental (Negative)
(Love) Emotional (Fear)
(Health) Physical (Disease)

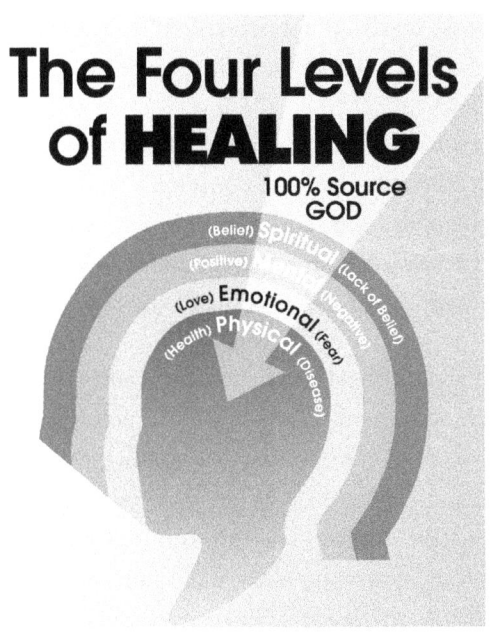

The Four Levels of Healing

Notice that healing starts at the top (God-source) and flows down through the body's different layers. Every negative block of energy caused by negative emotions, disempowering beliefs and thoughts diminish healing of the physical body.

The emotional level of healing is the closest to the physical realm. Trapped, or repressed emotions, are involved in every disease. These emotions are remnants of negative experiences from childhood, which are "stuck" in the body, causing a lower, slower, and sicker body. These "low frequency bundles of negative energy" are usually subconscious, so you don't even realize they are hiding deep in the darkness of your mind. Just because you don't know they are there, doesn't stop the damage being done. These "energy terrorists" are self-sabotaging your life. Muscle testing can locate and release subconscious, negative emotions. Refer to Chapter 17 for more information about emotional treatment programs.

Many natural health practitioners agree the number one cause of cancer is repressed, hidden emotions. Negative emotions make the body too acidic. Every feeling, whether it is love, or fear, causes a reaction in every cell. A positive, loving emotion creates a life-giving energy, that heals the cell. A negative, fearful emotion sends a message to every cell of doom and destruction. Which one do you think is going to make you healthier?

When a person is sick and goes to the doctor, emotional causes are never discussed. To truly heal the conscious, and subconscious, harmful emotions must be addressed, and released. The great news is these energy disruptors can be removed. Years of negative "junk" can be eliminated, and you can be freed from the demons of the past.

The mental level of healing affects your emotional state. The mental realm is formed by what you believe, and how you think. How you perceive the world, what you believe and how you think controls how you feel. The Bible states "as a man *thinketh* so is he." Everything starts with a thought. If you have a negative, disempowering, thought you send disruption, and lower energy throughout your body which creates stress, and imbalance eventually resulting in disease. Every positive, empowering, thought builds a stronger mind, body and soul. Be more aware of your thoughts. Thoughts are things that create health or disease. For more information on the mental realm of healing refer to my book *Resurrecting Your Life*.

The spiritual level of healing is the highest level of healing, It affects all of the other levels. It is also the most misunderstood, as far as healing is concerned. To truly heal, a person needs to awaken to the truth about the concept of God. The teachings of religions about a vengeful, angry, super human, God watching over our every move, and sending us to hell, is totally wrong. God is love. Love is healing. Fear is not healing. A spiritual, not religious, belief and attitude is crucial for abundant health.

To understand the importance of the spiritual aspects of healing is to understand who you truly are. This is the most important part of the healing process, and because of our toxic religious training, it is the hardest to convey, We are made in the image of God. We are God's creation. Our bodies are working miracles. Our bodies are the temple of God. God is not out there somewhere. God is within each of us. This creative energy is ever present and everywhere. If that is true, and I believe it is, then where does that place illness? Remember: God is not sick!

There is an order of divine guidance that controls how energy flows through the body. Any where there is a "block" of negative energy, in any level of healing, it stops the vital life force to flow into that particular tissue, organ or gland.

John, a pastor of a large congregation, and his wife, came to see me for an appointment. His wife had brought him to the office because she was concerned about his health. At the third appointment, I could tell that John was different - angry. I asked him what was wrong. He told me that he was "firing" me, because I had not made him any better. I agreed with him that he wasn't any better, and since this was the last time I was going to see him, I wanted to share with him the truth of why he wasn't getting better.

I showed him the Four Levels of Healing diagram. I looked the pastor in the eyes and asked, "what is your relationship with God?" Being a pastor, I thought that it would be an easy question for such a "Godly" man, but the answer I received was shocking.

"I'm mad at God," he answered. "He has placed too much responsibility on me." That scored -25% of the four levels of healing.

I thought to myself, how big of ego this man had, but continued my questioning. "Do you think positive or negative?" Again, assuming a strong, positive response, I heard him say "about 80% - 20%" which I answered "that's pretty good."

But, he quickly corrected my erroneous assumption, "80% negative!" Again, another -25% deducted from his four levels of healing.

Moving to the third question, I asked the pastor, "How are your emotions? Are you at peace? Do you focus on love or fear?"

"I'm always in fear;" he quickly exclaimed. Here he was sitting in front of me with a body at least fifty pounds overweight. He wasn't taking care of the temple that he supposedly believed in.

This "religious" man scored a 0%. He failed all four levels of healing, but was blaming me, as if I wasn't doing my job, getting him healthy. He did not want to take responsibility for his own health. He didn't have the desire, or the drive to find the road to true health. To regain your health, you must take responsibility.

The highest vibration of pure "white light" energy is the Universal All-Knowing Presence that many of us call God. God is pure love. God is pure energy. God is not sick, because God has no false ideas or beliefs. God is perfect health.

Looking at the diagram, imagine drawing a straight line from the word God (the abundant supply of health), which is pure healing energy, straight through the spiritual, mental and emotional planes, landing in the physical body. Without any blockages caused by religious toxic beliefs, negative thoughts, fear-based emotions, or nutritional deficiencies, the body would receive this pure, healing energy instantly. It would be like heaven. You wouldn't feel any pain. You would have a healthy body. You would be healed, but…

This beautiful, healing vibration, from the source of love that God is always giving us, is always flowing. But, what happens is this healing energy gets blocked by negative, false beliefs locked in the spiritual, mental, and emotional levels of our being. These disruptions of energy are disempowering beliefs, negative thoughts, past programming and life experiences. There is so much static that the message of love which heals isn't able to be received by the physical body. This Godly, healing energy, is always there for us, just like the rays of the sun. Negative thoughts and feelings are like a cloudy day that blocks the rays of the sun.

Every trapped emotion, or disempowering belief, distorts this energy flow. This disrupted energy travels through each layer, and the physical body receives the "altered" energy. This "altered" energy is not the energy that the Creator sent to the body. It has been blocked, much like an eclipse of the sun. The pure, loving energy, which is the healing energy, is always shining, but when it has been negatively influenced through the filtration of the mind, it changes into a lower vibration which is not healing.

As I stated earlier, muscle testing is one of the best tools to test subtle energy. Knowing about the four levels of healing, I believe you will understand the only way to find the root cause of most health conditions requires muscle testing. Muscle testing can find these self-sabotaging blockages of stagnate energy in these invisible energy levels, and remove them using energy medicine techniques.

As a society, we are addressing health care "backasswards." When there is a physical health problem most people visit a medical doctor, which is going to do an exam only on the physical level. But, as the diagram illustrates, the effect in the body doesn't begin in the physical area where they are examining. Illness or perfect health form in the invisible realms, long before it is manifested into the physical body. Yes, the physical area needs to be addressed, but there are always deeper issues that are not being considered, and the medical equipment cannot test. To truly heal, you must learn how to test all levels of healing via muscle testing.

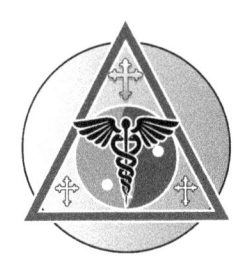

CHAPTER FOUR

The Art and Science of Muscle Testing

"I feel sorry for people who can't muscle test."
Dr. James Overmann (founder of Precision Herbs)

I still remember the day I was introduced to muscle testing. A friend of mine introduced me to a lady who was the leader of a multilevel marketing company. As a busy hairdresser with a large clientele, they wanted me to join their sales group. I wasn't interested, until this lady muscle tested me to "prove" to me that I needed their product. At first, I thought the demonstration was some type of trick. I was intrigued more about the muscle testing, than the product. I bargained with them that I would join their group, if she taught me how to muscle test.

For the next six months, I followed this lady to her other meetings, watching, and learning this skill, eventually helping her test the multitudes of people who wanted to be muscle tested. Once I was confident of my muscle testing skills, we departed ways, and I launched out on my own.

I had a built-in hairdressing clientele, so I started there. I would offer a free muscle testing demonstration to any client who was interested. At this time, I muscle tested people to see if they needed a certain product or not, and that was the start of my muscle testing career.

Things have changed over the last twenty years. The Body Balance Healing System was created from this first concept of muscle testing – if the product is beneficial for the body, the arm stays strong. If the chosen supplement is not beneficial for the body, the arm goes weak. Learning that the innate intelligence of the body "knew" what was beneficial and non-beneficial for the body, I started asking questions about the anatomy of the body. I discovered that I could ask any question, and the body's higher intelligence would answer a "yes," or "no". The Body Balance Healing System, which is the program taught in this book, is now advanced enough to find imbalances in the blood, tissue or cell. Over the years, many of these finding have been confirmed by blood tests, and most importantly - improvement in people's personal health.

I understand that some people will be skeptical about muscle testing. If you are skeptical, I don't blame you. I was very skeptical when I was first shown muscle testing. I was convinced that it was some type of trick. So, I did the only thing I could do to prove that it was true or not, and that was I learned how to muscle test. You really can't fully understand the concept, or the art, without learning it yourself.

After lots of practice, I started feeling confident, and I was hooked. When the "aha" moment struck me that I could now communicate with the body, and learn whatever I ask, it was a whole, new, unlimited world, to explore. Yes, I made mistakes, but I continued learning, and feeling more and more confident.

Years later, I had a patient call me, complaining that I had made a mistake, and given her the wrong supplement. I listened to her story, as she explained how she had done her own research on the supplements, and after reading the company information. there was nowhere in the information stating that this particular supplement was designed to do what I was using it for. I agreed with her, and then asked the confused lady if I could ask her one question –"Do *you* muscle test?" She answered with a surprised "no." I informed her as nicely as I could, but firmly, "you can't understand what I am doing, if you don't muscle test." I believe that is true for every person.

Learning how to muscle test changed my life. Every member of my family has benefited from muscle testing. They all believe in the power it has to connect to the ultimate truth. This next story will share the feelings of trust that my family shares about muscle testing.

Our son, Michael, who is also a Naturopath doctor, was fixing a special dinner for the family. He had prepared sweet potatoes, and right before we were getting ready to sit down and eat, he decided to pour maple syrup over the potatoes. To the family's shock, the syrup was full of mold. To everyone else, the plate would have been ruined – but not Michael. He had just ruined his potatoes, but he didn't give up. He washed, and cleaned each potato, and then muscle tested each potato for it being safe to eat and free of mold or mold toxins.. He informed us that all the sweet potatoes muscle tested safe and free of mold. We blessed the food, and ate every bite with no hesitation! That is putting your life in the hands of muscle testing!

I have had my current position as the Naturopathic doctor at Health and Wellness of Carmel (www.hwofc.com) for the last eight years because of muscle testing. The owner, Dr. Cliff Fetters, had been hearing my name from his patients, who were coming to see me between their office visits with him. He noticed that the patients, who were also seeing me, were getting healthier. He decided to find out for himself about what I was doing.

The receptionist informed me my last patient, that evening, was Dr. Cliff Fetters – an MD making an appointment with me. He was the first medical doctor I had ever tested. The appointment went well, and after a few visits, he informed me that I was "the real thing", and he invited me to join his integrative medical practice. It was like going from the minor league, to playing with one of the best teams in the major leagues.

The other MD in the practice wasn't so sure about my muscle testing skills. He decided that he would challenge me. Both of the doctors had just completed a $700 DNA exam. As this skeptical doctor held his exam in his hand, he challenged me by asking if muscle testing could tell him the same results. I accepted the challenge, knowing absolutely nothing about DNA. He handed me the twenty-five blank questions, hiding the blood test results. I started the exam by muscle testing the doctor for each of the twenty-five categories. Within each category there were three options – 0%; 50%; or 100%. I didn't understand what the differences were, but continued testing, as the doctor recorded my answers. After I finished, he compared my answers to the computer results. In total disbelief, he informed me that I was 100% correct!

After hearing about what I had done, Dr. Fetters wanted me to do his DNA exam in front of the entire staff. I did the same exam, and scored 95%. The doctors were impressed. Patients are impressed, Muscle testing is real. It is one of the most accurate "diagnostic" tools available, for not only professionals, but every person who takes the time to learn.

This is how confident I hope you become with muscle testing. Every person who is willing, can learn this valuable "life style" tool. You will get out of it exactly what you put into it. Don't worry, if you don't first catch on. Just keep practicing. Find the one technique that you feel you are the best at, and practice that one until you master it. Practice everywhere you go. Play a game. Make a statement and test. Make an obvious statement, such as the color of the car next to you, or the day of the week, and test for strong. Once you master the true response, change to a false statement, and make a statement, or question, about the color of the car next to you that is false or the wrong day of the week and practice feeling false.

Please don't tell yourself, or others that you "can't do it." This skill is too valuable to just give up on. My mentor, Dr. James Overman once said, "I feel sorry for people who can't muscle test." I agree. I suggest to all of our patients to learn how to muscle test. Don't lose this chance to have something so unique, and practical, that you can use the rest of your life. Just, understand that it is going to take practice, persistence, practice, patience and more practice. You will go through a time that you believe you are controlling the test. Don't worry. This too shall pass.

Use this book as your muscle testing manual. Don't just read it. Use it. Everything it takes to be a great muscle tester is in this book.

What is Muscle Testing?

Before we go into the techniques of muscle testing, lets understand exactly what muscle testing is, how it works, and then learn the fundamentals of muscle testing. By learning the foundational concepts of this art will make understanding the program easier.

As I have already stated, the body is electric. This flow of energy is not physical, and cannot be measured by standard medical equipment. Every tissue of your body has to have a good energy flow to be healthy. The body's intelligence system knows precisely what is going on in your body. If the energy flow of a particular area of the body's energy is not perfect, that particular organ, or gland, will be weaker than normal.

When this particular organ, or gland, is named, and the muscle tested, the muscle will go weak. Whenever the muscle goes weak, electrical flow is not correct, because of some type of imbalance.

Here's how it works. When the body's electrical system is flowing correctly, the resistance of the muscle will test strong. But, if the electric system is damaged, and has a short circuit, then the reaction of the muscle, when tested, will go weak. This is not because of the strength of the tester, or lack of physical strength of the person being tested. The lack of resistance of the muscle signifies a short circuit in the electrical system, caused by an imbalance of energy in the body. Once this imbalance is corrected, the circuit is repaired, and the flow of lifeforce energy is restored. The muscle being tested can now resist the tester's pressure, showing no more weakness in that area - indicating good energy flow which creates optimum health.

To be healthy, the body must be in balance (homeostasis). This balance is achieved when all systems are functioning perfectly. Health is more than just the absence of disease. This concept of perfect balance should be an on- going lifetime journey of keeping yourself, and your loved ones, as healthy as possible for as long as possible. By learning muscle testing, and using the Body Balance Healing System you can do that.

The FUNdamentals of Muscle Testing

Here are some basic concepts that must be learned to muscle test correctly. By understanding these foundational concepts, your experience of muscle testing will be more rewarding. The Body Balance Healing System teaches muscle testing differently than other programs. Some concepts and techniques are similar, but there are important differences, which can make a huge difference in the accuracy and results.

The first muscle testing technique is the "arm" test. To use this technique there must be two people present – you being the tester, and a person being tested (testee). The following objectives must be considered before starting the test.

1. Sitting position for the testee, and the tester
2. Arm position for the testee/ hand position for tester
3. Polarity

Testing Positions

When you are muscle testing another person, make sure that these positions are correct. If both of you are sitting, you should sit facing each other. Make sure that both sets of feet are on the ground – not crossed. The tester should be sitting slightly higher than the testee. This provides better leverage during the testing. Remember, muscle testing is NOT a strength test, but rather a resistance test. It is not as tiring on the tester if you have a height advantage.

Both you and the person you are testing can stand and test. This does get tiring, so I suggest sitting. The results will be the same. If you are testing someone who is bigger and stronger than you, have the testee to sit and you stand. As long as you follow all of the steps, either sitting or standing will work.

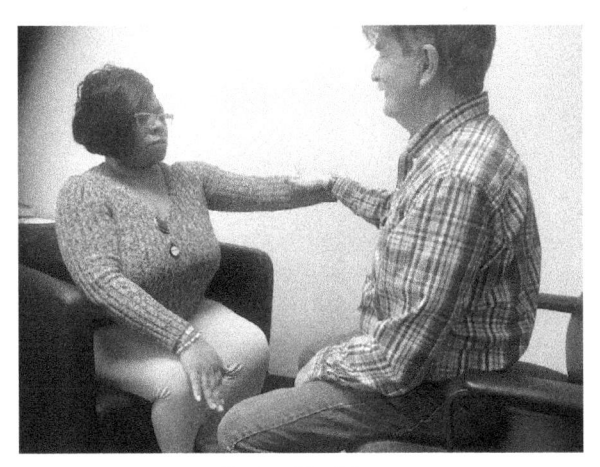

Sitting Position

This is the most popular testing position. Ask the person being tested to uncross their legs and keep both feet on the floor for better testing. Ask the person to remove their watch, magnets and jewelry that might create disturbance in the energy field.

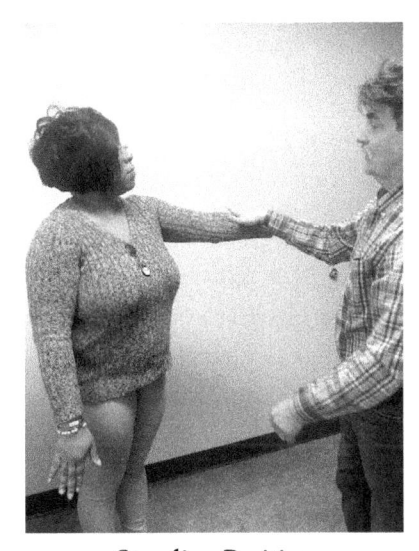

Standing Position

Both the tester and testee standing is the least used position. It is tiring for both involved. There is no advantage to standing and testing. If the tester believes that the standing position is better, it can be used and the results are the same. The standing position is not the same as the sway technique, which is a muscle testing procedure that the person stands quietly while holding the supplement. If the body sways forward it is a positive response. If the body falls backwards the answer is no. This technique is not taught in this system.

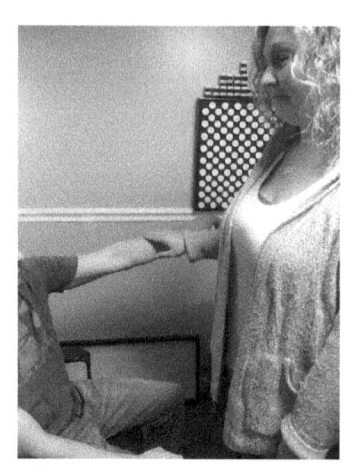

Subject Sitting/Tester Standing

This is a "power" position to get extra leverage for the tester. It is never the intention to overpower the subject, but there are times when this position is very useful. This position is perfect when the person being tested is stronger than the tester. An example might be a female tester trying to test a body builder or football player. It does require applying pressure on the arm to evaluate the response so the extra leverage can be helpful and not as tiring

Arm Testing

One of the differences in this program, from other muscle testing programs, is the position of the testing arm. Either the right or left arm can be used, as long as there is no pain or physical injury. Ask the testee if there are any weakness, or pain in their shoulder, arm, elbow, wrist, or hand. If there is a problem, you will have to either use the other arm, if it is healthy, or one of the one hand muscle testing techniques, you will be learning. The subject being tested will hold their arm horizontal to the floor. This does get tiring, so inform the person to put their arm down when you are not testing them.

Besides being horizontal to the floor, the arm should be positioned at 45 degrees. To find this angle, consider straight out in front of the person 0 degree, and the arm out from the shoulder 90 degrees (normal position for most muscle testing programs). The correct position is in the middle of these two positions, which is 45 degrees. Determined through muscle testing, this position of the arm is the only angle that tests all meridians.

(See picture). The last thing that the person being tested must do is to lock the elbow.

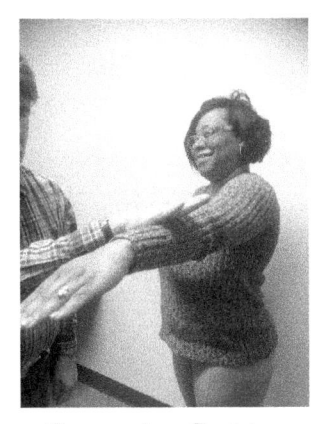

Correct Arm Position

If you consider holding your arm straight out in front of you is 0 and holding it straight out to your side being 90 degrees, the correct arm position is 45 degrees (exactly in the middle of those two positions.) This is important because the mostly widely used – the 90 degree position does not test all meridians. The 45 degree tests all meridians. The arm should be held firm with the hand open and fingers straight. The arm should be held horizontal to the floor. Testing can be done on whichever arm is the strongest.

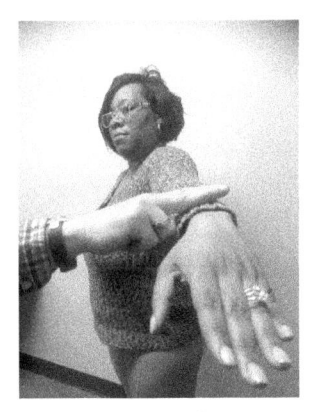

Incorrect Arm Position

This is the 90 degree position that many muscle testers use. Through muscle testing it can be proven that this 90% position of the arm does *not* test the energy of *all* of the meridians. Muscle test by asking "Does the 90 degree arm position correctly test the energy of *all* meridians?" Then ask, "Does the 45 degree arm position correctly test *all* meridians?" By asking these two questions and accurately muscle testing you will know the truth.

You, the tester, will place your open hand, palm down on the testee's outstretched arm. Placement should be your palm is flat against the other persons forearm, between the wrist and the elbow, but closer to the wrist. (See picture).

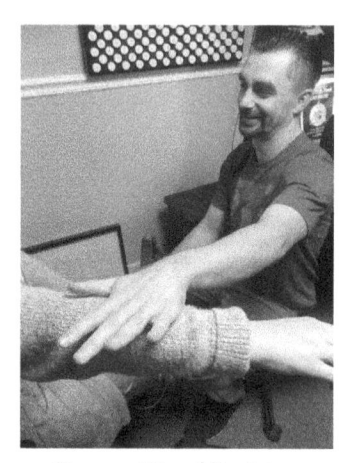

Correct Hand Position

The open palm of the testing hand is placed across the lower forearm of the subject. If the right arm is being used the tester will use the left hand. If the left arm is used the right hand should be used. Notice that the palm is placed closer to the wrist than the elbow but not on the wrist. This is not the best.

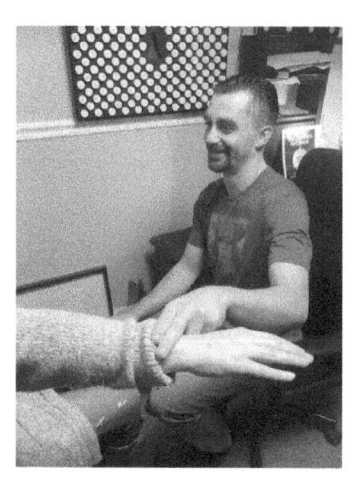

Incorrect Hand Position

Notice that two fingers are being used on the wrist. This testing procedure, used by many muscle testers, encourage "flipping" of the wrist which creates an inaccurate muscle testing.

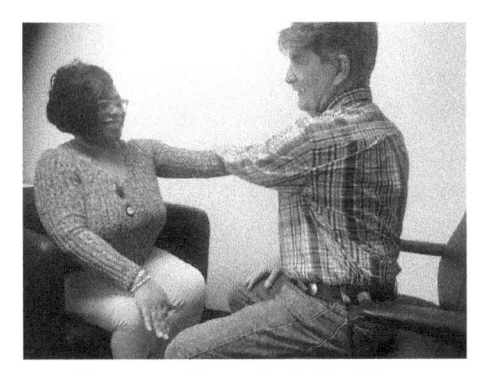

Incorrect Cross Body Position

Never cross your arm across the body during testing. This blocks the energy flow which could give false or inaccurate testing.

Another difference in this system from other muscle testing procedures is the placement of your hand when testing the arm. Many muscle testers do the resistance test on the wrist. We believe this area is too weak, and flimsy, to do an accurate test. If you think of the arm as the lever you want it strong. By moving between the wrist and the elbow, slightly closer to the wrist, this is a much better test.

Also, many muscle testers use only two fingers on the wrist, which can create too much "wrist action". By using the whole opened hand, you achieve a slow, smooth, even pressure, when you perform the muscle test. Some people will challenge you, by claiming that you pushed harder on the weak response. Slow, steady, even pressure, on every statement or question, is your goal to become an accurate muscle tester.

What you don't want to do is to rush muscle testing. The body needs a moment to respond. When testing, after you make the statement, or question, wait a few seconds, then test. You will receive a more accurate answer. I have seen testers try to receive the answer from the body, almost before they finished the statement.

Remember, muscle testing is not a strength test. Your job is not to "win" by forcing their arm down. Muscle testing is to find the truth. Muscle testing can do that, if the muscle test is performed correctly.

The "lock" involves the deltoid muscles, located at the top of the shoulder. This area is called the "lock" because when a question or statement is true, the deltoid muscles, of the person being tested, will stay strong against the pressure. But, when a question or statement is false or harmful to the body, these same muscles will not be able to resist the slight resistance and won't lock firm.

When you apply pressure against the subject's outstretched arm, you will be able to feel whether the muscle locks, and the arm stays strong, or the muscle doesn't lock, and the arm will not be able to resist the downward pressure.

The answer is in the "lock". When people watch muscle testing, most watch the arm, but that is not where the answer is hidden. Imagine the arm as a lever, and the deltoid muscles the fulcrum. The answer is whether the muscle locks or don't lock in the shoulder area. It is a lie detector for the body, detecting true, or false What's wonderful about this locking mechanism is that after only a few well executed muscle tests, the testee will be able to feel whether their shoulder locks in and gets strong or goes weak. At this point, they are starting to learn the language of the body and how to communicate with it. That's what muscle testing does.

Starting To Muscle Test

Now that you have learned the starting positions of both you and the person that you are testing, it's time to actually start muscle testing. The first step is to verify the person you are testing is strong enough to be tested. After placing the testee's arm in the correct position, request the testee to "hold firm." Wait a few seconds, and then slowly, start a smooth downward, resistance against the person's outstretched arm. If the subject can hold their arm up against the pressure, then they are strong enough to test. If one arm is too weak, try the other arm. If both arms are too weak, the first reason is possibly dehydration. Have them either drink water or place a water bottle against their body, and then test again. If water doesn't improve the situation, then you will need to select another method of muscle testing, such as surrogate or one hand testing.

If the person passes the first test, the next step is confirming the testee and your polarity is correct. What is polarity? It is the flow of energy in the body. When polarity is correct, the body answers strong to truth and weak for false. If polarity is reversed, then every answer is wrong and the opposite of what is actually true. True questions would muscle test weak, false questions tests strong.

I personally know how important polarity is because I have experienced the effects of not checking polarity. A patient had an appointment with me in the morning. As always, I started my exam by testing polarity, and everything was fine. I did my exam and she finished. Later that day, she called the office in a panic, telling me she had just returned from her chiropractor visit, and he told her that she needed to get to the hospital because she was getting ready to have a heart attack! She was in a panic, and called me to see what I thought. I told her to come over immediately, and I would work her in my already busy schedule.

Rushing her in, I started doing the exam, and it looked like the chiropractor was right. Everything I checked in the heart was testing weak! I freaked out, and confirmed what the other doctor said, and she rushed over to the hospital to find out there was nothing wrong. I questioned how in the world I could have been so wrong, and then I figured it out. I had not established her polarity the second visit. I assumed that she was still in polarity but this shocking news from her chiropractor, threw her out of polarity, and all my testing was opposite and wrong. That is how important checking polarity every time – even if you see them more than once per day.

To confirm polarity, state questions or statements that are universal truths, and universal falsehoods. By doing this, you are confirming that the arm stays strong when a truth is spoken, and it goes weak when the statement or question is untrue. Start with an obvious truth such as 2 + 2 = 4. Make the statement, "Two plus two is four." You can ask the question, 'Does two plus two equal four?" You can state their name, such as "This is "the person's name." Wait a few seconds, and then gently push down on the testee's arm. The muscle/arm should stay strong. If it doesn't stay strong, the person is either out of polarity, too weak to test or it's the wrong name. The next test will tell you the answer.

The next part of testing polarity is testing for a negative response. This time you will make a statement that is false, such as 2 + 2 = 10. Another technique is state,"this is and use a wrong name." Questions can also be used, such as, "is this (wrong name)? Remember to pause for a few seconds after making the statement, or question, and then apply, smooth, even pressure to the arm. Either of these statements should make the arm go weak.

When a true statement tests weak, and a false statement tests strong, the person's polarity is out of balance. This must be corrected before you can proceed.

Correcting Polarity

The body's polarity is like a battery. If you put the batteries in a flashlight backwards, the flashlight will not work. The reason is, the batteries are in backwards. The flow of electrical energy can't work, when polarity is upside down. The human body is no different. When your polarity is not correct, the body can't give the correct answers through muscle testing.

The most common reason polarity gets switched to its opposite field is negative, emotional energy, and vibrations. A sudden, negative, emotional, experience can knock a person out of energetic balance. Another reason it happens is if a person is struck by lightning. The lightning's electrical charge reverses the body's polarity.

Now that you know what polarity is, and how important it is to accurately muscle test, let's learn how to correct a persons' polarity. I recommend two different techniques. You can choose which one you like, or use them both. I suggest doing the polarity correcting exercise every day, whether you need it or not. The practice takes only a few minutes, won't hurt you if you don't need it, and starts your day in a better vibration.

The Thymus Thump

Donna Eden, the mother of energy work, introduced the Thymus Thump exercise in her book, *Energy Medicine*. The thymus gland is the major gland of the immune system. It is located in the middle area of your breastbone (where Tarzan beat on his chest and did his jungle yell). To perform the Thymus Thump, continually tap the sternum area, with your fingertips, or knuckles, as you breathe a deep breath. Keep thumping, until you have finished three deep breaths. (See picture)

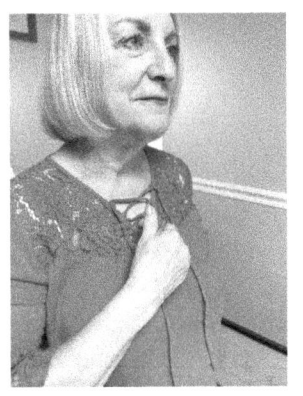

The Thymus Thump

This technique is used to correct polarity when polarity is reversed. To correct polarity, have the person being tested to continue tapping the thymus gland and doing three deep breaths while tapping. Three times will realign the polarity, which is imperative for accurate muscle testing. It is a good idea for the tester to do the thymus tap on themselves before testing to make sure that both people are in polarity. The tester can do the thymus thump on the subject if desired by the patient but it is better for the person to get involved.

The Zipper Method

Picture zipping up your jacket. Do this motion with your hand open, and palm facing the body, but not touching the person. With your open hand, continue moving up the zipper line, all the way through the middle of the face, middle of the forehead and finish at the back of the head, near the nape. The line that you just "traced" with the palm of your hand, is called the Governing Meridian in Chinese medicine. The palm of your hand has an electromagnetic quality, which is healing to the body. Perform this "zipping" three times, while doing deep breaths. (See picture).

Once you complete one, or both of these exercises, retest for polarity. If the person is testable, then polarity will be corrected.

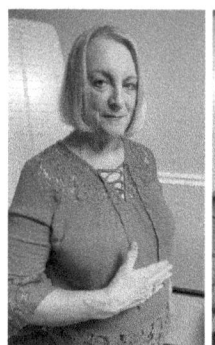

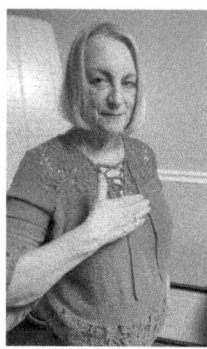

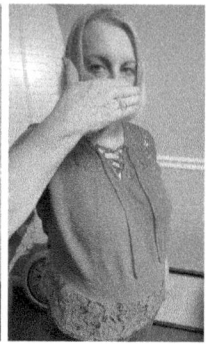

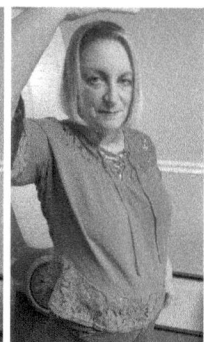

The Zipper Method

Another method to correct polarity is the zipper method. Place your open palm close to the pelvic area (9A) and start moving your open hand up the middle front of the body (9B) as if zipping up a jacket. Continue moving up and finish at the bridge of the nose. (9C) With this technique, the tester or testee can perform it. You do not have to touch the body for this to work. This technique is correcting energy flow. By staying within an inch or two of the body you are still in the subject's aura (energy field). CAUTION: By swiping down the body from the chin down to the pelvic area disrupts the energy field and will negatively affect polarity.

Other Muscle Testing Techniques

Surrogate Testing

Once you master arm testing, you can do surrogate testing. Surrogate testing is using the arm of a third person to muscle test someone who is not strong enough to personally be tested. When you only know how to arm test, and you want to muscle test a baby, disabled/ill person, who doesn't have the energy to hold their arm strong or a pet surrogate testing is perfect.

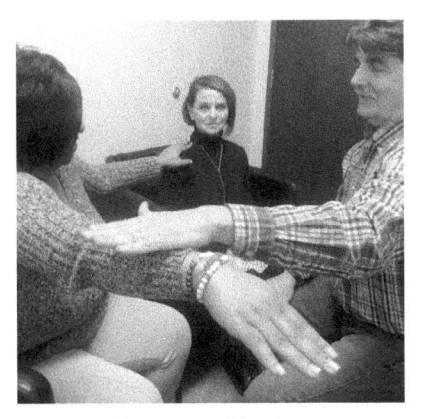

Surrogate Testing

If a person is present, but unable to be personally tested and arm testing is the only method known, surrogate testing is a perfect solution. Once one hand testing is learned surrogate testing is not necessary. The difference of surrogate testing and remote testing is that surrogate testing is using a third party's arm to get answers for the other non-testable person who is present. Remote testing is testing a person who is not physically with the tester.

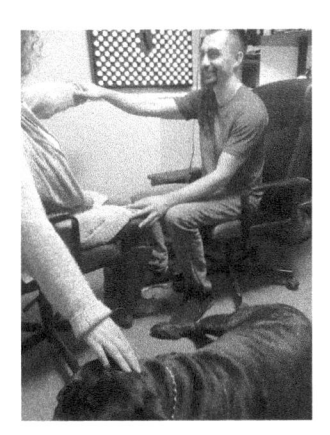

Surrogate Testing For Pets

Surrogate testing works perfectly for pets. They are actually easier to heal because in most cases they don't have the negative beliefs, thoughts and emotions that are blocking the flow of energy for naturally healing.

To perform surrogate testing, first test the person who's arm you will be using for the testing (the surrogate). Confirm polarity. Once that is established, "connect" the surrogate to the person, or pet you desire to test by touching each other. Once contact is made, insure you are testing the correct energy by ask;

Is this (subject's name) energy?"

If the body answers, "yes," ask;

"Is this (the surrogate's name) energy?"

This question should test false, signaling a "no" response. If the question is true, the connection has not been made. Repeat the questions with more intent, and focus on who you are testing. Once the first question is true, and the second is false you are ready to establish polarity of the person you are testing.

If polarity is correct the testing can begin, but if it isn't correct, perform the thymus thump, or zipper technique, on the person being tested, not the surrogate.

Once you learn one hand muscle testing, you won't need to use surrogate testing, unless you have a third party, who wants to see "proof."

Using the indicator arm as your tool for muscle testing is great, but there are some drawbacks. There are times, and situations that arm testing is not possible, such as remote testing Then what do you do? Don't worry. There are other options that you have to choose from. One downside of arm testing is that you can't test yourself. What if the person is too weak, and you can't use their arm? What about wanting to test a baby? You can't test your pets, with arm testing. How about testing somebody, that is long distance from you? The good news is, there are many different techniques you can use to muscle test. You can experiment, and find which one you feel the most confident. Start with what feels most comfortable, and use that technique, until you have mastered that one. Once you have accomplished the first technique, you can explore another technique. Learn as many as possible, and use them all in your toolbelt of natural health.

Table Top Testing

I don't personally use this technique, but because it is taught in our Muscle Testing 101 class, I wanted to share it with you. This technique is a perfect way to start testing without using the arm. It is a good choice, if you are having trouble picking up the other options. I learned this muscle testing technique from an MD who uses it in his practice. It has been used successfully by our students, as they get more comfortable with the other techniques.

To use the *Table Top* technique, place one of your hands on a flat surface, palm side down. Lift your index finger of that hand. This finger is the indicator muscle, which you use to muscle test. (see photo below). Hold your finger firmly, off the surface, in a horizontal position, as if it was the arm. Use the index finger of your opposite hand, and place it on top of the indicator finger. Apply slight pressure against it while your outstretched finger resists the pressure. Just like the arm, if the indicator finger stays strong against the pressure, the answer is true. If the finger goes weak, it is false.

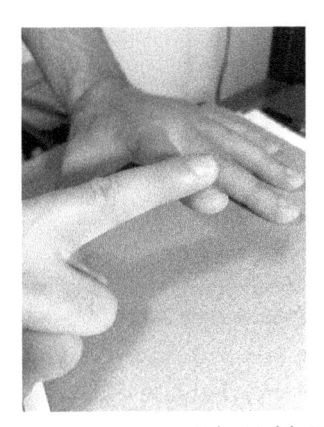

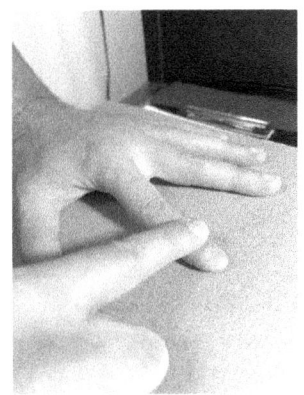

The Table Top Method

This technique is the easiest of all the hand testing techniques. It still takes two hands. This technique is taught in our muscle testing classes because it gives every student an easy, simple technique to start doing "independent" muscle testing (you don't have to have someone else's arm to test something or someone). The Table Top method can be done right or left-handed.

One Hand Techniques
The Two Finger Technique

The following two techniques are the most popular, besides the arm test. The first of these two starts with the index finger, or middle finger held horizontally. If you are holding the index finger horizontally, place your middle finger on top of the index finger pressing at the first knuckle. (see photo below) If you are holding your middle finger horizontally, you will place your index finger on top, placing the pressure at the first joint. (see photo) By applying pressure with the finger on top, you can judge whether the bottom finger stays strong or weak. The "lock" for these techniques is the joint that connects the finger to the hand.

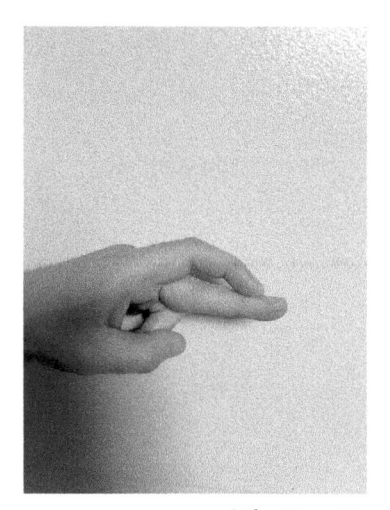

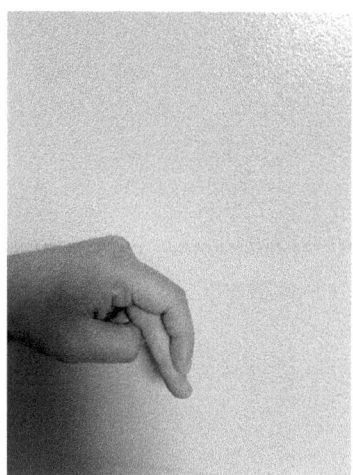

The Two Finger Technique

There are two options to this method. This first option is using the middle finger as the "arm." Hold the middle finger horizontal and strong. Place the index finger of the same hand on top of the middle finder touching the first knuckle. By pressing down on the middle finger with the index finger you can test for true or false, just like the arm. If the middle finger stays strong it is true and if it goes weak it signals false.

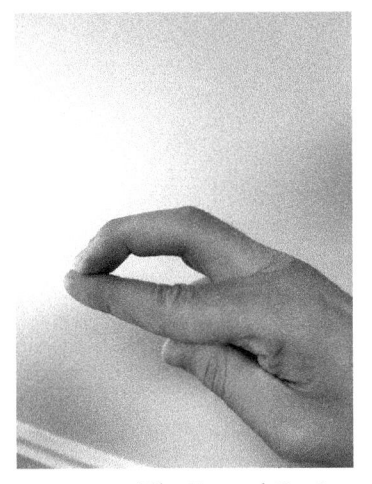

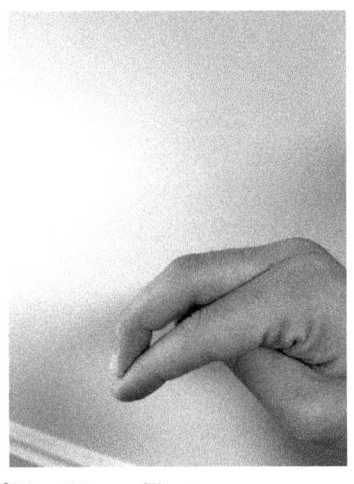

The Second Option of Two Finger Testing

This technique is the same except it uses the index finger as the arm and placing the middle finger on top of the index finger. Since the middle finger is longer than the index finger, this option gives more leverage. Both are as accurate as muscle testing with the arm once you master it. Both of these techniques can be done right or left-handed.

The Slide Technique

This technique is our most popular choice. Every person learning muscle testing, wants to learn this skill. Use the thumb and index finger and make a circle, with the thumb on the inner, top of the index finger. (see photo below) Press down enough that you can feel friction between the thumb and index fingers. Make it light enough so you don't place too much pressure, but enough to feel a difference. By putting pressure against your thumb, you should feel a resistance against the skin of the thumb. When this resistance stops your finger from sliding down, it indicates a strong "yes" answer.

When you apply the correct pressure, and the skin seems to get smooth, your index finger will not be able to stick. This is the indication of a false statement or question.

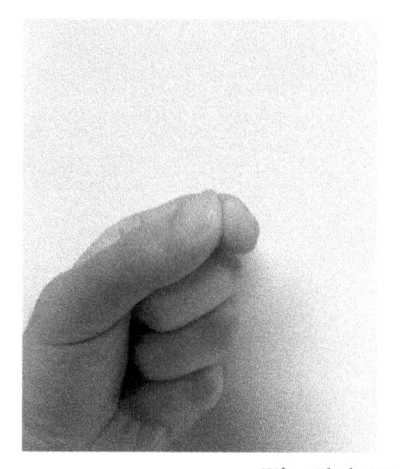

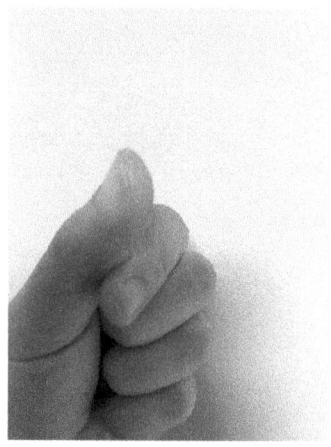

The Slide Technique

This method of muscle testing is the most desired and for many people the hardest to master. This is the technique that I personally use but incorporate two finger testing in my practice. To do the slide technique use the thumb and index finger or ring finger. Both are acceptable. Do not use the thumb and the middle finger. Press the thumb and fingers together to just feel a slight friction. When you try to slide your thumb past the index finger it "sticks." This signals a true answer. Again, pressing the thumb and finger together with the same pressure but the fingers slide apart, not having any friction. That is what false feels like. The false response is harder to feel but once you have it you will have it forever. This technique takes the most practice, patience and persistence to conquer, but once you master it you will never go back.

You now know all of the muscle testing techniques, that you will need to be a master muscle tester. There are others, such as the sway technique, but we don't teach it. It is okay for beginners, but it's too slow, and hard to be as accurate. Invest in your time, learning the techniques that we have discussed, and with practice, you will become a good muscle tester.

Remote or Distance Testing

Once you have learned how to finger test, you will be able to do remote testing. Remote testing is muscle testing a person, or pet, who are not at the same location. This is a valuable tool because it gives you the ability to help people anywhere in the world!

For some people, remote testing is hard to believe. They don't understand the concept of energy, that we are all connected in an electric field. The quantum physics concept, energy follows thought, supports this procedure.

There are many methods of remote testing. The most used is voice. By talking on the phone, a good muscle tester can test the person through hearing the voice. With today's technical advancements, the tester and the person being tested can see each other through Zoom, and other social media platforms. With the onslaught of CoVid19 tele-visits have increased dramatically, and remote testing is now being used by medical doctors. The problem with medical doctors doing these remote exams is the doctor doesn't muscle test, so it is an educated guess.

Integrative functional medical doctor, Dr. Cliff Fetters, personally thanked me for us teaching him how to do finger testing. He was already arm testing, but finger testing opened up the world for his practice. His remote testing has increased, and getting better results, because he can now use his knowledge, and muscle testing together, to give his patients the best treatment that they deserve.

Remote testing is just as accurate as on-site testing. We do remote testing in practically every state. Many of these patients have been receiving remote tests for years, and continue because they are getting results. Remote testing works.

Congratulations! At this time, you have now finished the first level as a beginning muscle tester. Now, it is up to you to practice as much as you can. To improve your finger muscle testing skills, muscle test everything around you. Make statements about a color of car or sign. Make a negative statement such as stating "the car next to me is red." If the car is actually red, then your finger should stay strong, but if the car is actually white, then it should go weak. You can ask questions or make statements about whatever you notice while sitting at the stoplight. (Don't worry. If you get engrossed in your testing, and not paying attention to the green light, the person behind you will quickly let you know). Here are just some of the things that you will now be able to muscle test;

1. You can test if a food is beneficial. All you do is hold the actual food against the body, and see if the muscle tests strong or weak. You don't have to eat it. If it stays strong, that food is beneficial. If it goes weak, it is not a healthy choice. If the food, or supplement, is not available, just saying the name of the food, or supplement, without actually having it physically in your hand, will test the same as if it was present. The universal, All-Knowing energy of God, and the intelligence of the body knows..
2. You can test what supplements your body needs, and how many you need. Again, either hold the supplement, or say the name of the supplement, and test for strong or weak,
3. You can use your imagination and test anything you desire.

In my past I have seen muscle testing used for many things. One of our muscle testing students had lost her pet snake. She asked me about it. We muscle tested that "Gertrude" was still in the house. I instructed the young lady to go to her house, stand inside the front door, and test which direction she should go to find her pet. She called me back within a half hour, telling me she had found her baby through muscle testing.

Another example, and one that I would not suggest, was one of the students of muscle testing for years, felt that her husband was cheating on her. She asked me if she could muscle test if it was true. My answer was that universal energy, which muscle testing connects to, knows all. I suggested for her not to do it, but she did anyway. She discovered her husband *was* cheating on her. And she did it completely through trusting muscle testing. The husband finally did admit that he was cheating on her. Muscle testing brought out the truth and yes, in this instance the truth did set her free.

You can't use muscle testing to pick lottery numbers, predict the future, card playing or any type of gambling. I also would not suggest using it to make major life decisions. Muscle testing is a God-given gift to help yourself, and others with their health. It's not for personal gain. It is to help you, and others restore health, and rebuild the body. Health is wealth. By keeping yourself healthy, you can be a shining example, and inspire others. Helping a person regain their health is an honor, and a privilege I don't take lightly. I hope you will feel the same way about the art of muscle testing.

Even if you stop after finishing Level I, muscle testing will help you in many ways. It takes practice, patience and persistence to trust your muscle testing skill, but the more you do it the better you will get. Don't be too hard on yourself. Some people pick it up faster than others. If you continue practicing, with a positive attitude, you will become a good muscle tester. You will be able to use it for the rest of your life, so if it takes you more time to learn the skill, it's okay. Relax and have fun with it.

You Can Heal – Naturally is designed in three levels. Once you are comfortable with your basic muscle testing skills, you can continue on to the second level, or stop and take a break. You can come back any time to review, or move into Level 2. If you decide you would like to keep going, and dive deeper into our program, it is time to move to Level 2 – Learning the Body Balance Healing System.

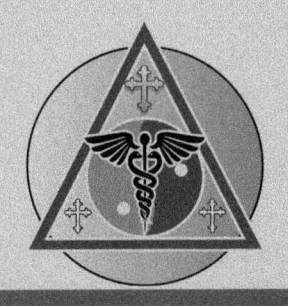

LEVEL 2

INTERMEDIATE

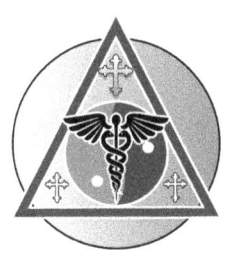

CHAPTER FIVE
The Body Balance Healing System

Now that you have learned the basic muscle testing techniques, it is time to find the root causes of your health issues. Many people know how to muscle test, but don't use an organized program to systematically locate the root cause. Most muscle testers can test what supplements you need. Few have a system they can muscle test as deep as the cell level. Multi-marketing companies use muscle testing to "sell" a potential customer they need the product. This procedure works, but is too general. This is why people consume too many supplements. A person can test strong on many products. The real question is, which exact supplements, or foods, are the best to correct the problem. Accurate muscle testing, combined with an organized system, will give you those answers. Please remember, all muscle testers are *not* created equal.

Using this system, combined with muscle testing, you will use only what you need to correct the current issue. By learning how to be more precise, instead of a general test, will save you money, time, and suffering, taking too many pills. The Body Balance Healing System is a better way. It is more precise, repeatable and logical. You will learn about the body's anatomy, and physiology. By communicating with your body, through the miracle of muscle testing, you can help your body heal naturally. If you use the steps below, you will soon be able to feel results. It has worked for thousands of patients and it will work for you.

Starting to Muscle Test

After establishing polarity, as discussed in Level 1, ask the body:

"Is this symptom (name your symptom) caused by a physical reason?"

If "yes", refer to The Body Balance Healing System Assessment Sheet in the Appendix. Start with the first system (circulatory), and continue down the list of the ten systems until you get a strong response (Yes). Ask;

"Is the first reason for this symptom in the circulatory system?"

If "no", continue down the list of systems; digestive system? intestinal system? … until you get a "yes" - a strong muscle resistance.

A strong response indicates the exact system where the first reason for the symptom is located. The next question is, where in that system is the problem located. Once you have located the system, move right along the choices in the selected system. Test each choice separately. A strong response indicates that this choice is where the root cause is located in that system.

An example; The circulatory system tests strong to the above question. Next you would proceed to the first option on that line to the right.

Circulatory__ Blood__ Heart__ Arteries__ Veins__ Capillaries__

"Is the first reason for this (your symptom) in the blood?"

If "no", go to the next choice to the right - heart?, arteries?, veins?... capillaries? Keep testing until one of the choices tests strong in the chosen system. Once you determine the system, where the root cause is located, there is a part in that system that is causing the problem. It's your job to find it, and you can do that via muscle testing.

Testing the Functioning of the Body

Once the specific part of the selected system is located, muscle test the percentage of functioning. Functioning is the measurement of how well, or poorly, an organ, gland, or tissue is functioning. When a system, organ, gland, tissue, or cell is functioning as God designed, it is working perfectly, and will never cause a problem or symptom. When the area is functioning perfectly, it will muscle test as 100%. If it's not functioning perfectly, the tester needs to determine the functioning percentage. If the area tests as 95% or higher (sufficiently) in most cases, it will not cause a symptom. Two organs that need to be perfect in functioning, are the brain and heart.

Muscle test for functioning by asking the following question;

"Is the organ, gland or tissue (in the area that you have located as the root cause) functioning at least sufficient?

If it tests strong (yes), then you haven't located the root cause yet. If you do have the correct location, the test question will go weak. This means that particular spot in the body is causing a problem because it is not functioning at least sufficiently. Next you need to determine the percentage of functioning.

If the above question tested weak (no) then start with the following question;

"Is this organ, gland or tissue (whatever you have designated as your root cause) functioning underactive?

If this question tests true, ask;

"Is the tissue, organ or gland functioning at least sufficiently?"

If "no", start by asking;

"Is this tissue functioning at least 90% or higher?"

If this question tests "no", continue decreasing by tens until the arm stays strong, confirming the area you are focused on is functioning at least at that number.

"Is this area working at 80? or higher, 70% or higher?"

YOU CAN HEAL NATURALLY • 53

The lower the functioning number, the worst the situation. You're always looking for the lowest, functioning number, based on 100%. Once you establish a base number of tens, you can test the exact functioning number. If the arm tests weak at 90% or higher, try 80% or higher, and continue until you get a strong response. Once you receive a strong muscle test, the following questions will guide you in determining the exact percentage of functioning. Assuming that 80% or higher tested strong, ask'

"Is the area functioning at 85% or better?"

If the muscle test stays strong, you know the functioning number is between 85% and 90%. If you want the exact number, start counting up from 85% (whatever number you have determined), and continue counting by two's until the muscle goes weak. The last strong test is your exact percentage of functioning. If you are a beginning muscle tester, the exact percentage of functioning isn't crucial.

Once the lowest functioning organ, gland or tissue has been determined, you can find out WHY this is happening, and WHAT you can do to correct it. This next section will give you the answers to the WHY and WHAT.

Testing For The WHY/WHAT?

All symptoms of ill health are caused by one thing – STRESS. There are four physical causes of stress, which create health problems. They are;

1. Toxins
2. Nutritional deficiencies
3. Parasites
4. Tissue damage

These four reasons are in the physical category of the Four Levels of Healing. The majority of symptoms tests in the physical realm. If you continue studying the system, you will learn about the emotional, mental, and spiritual aspects of healing.

Once you have located the specific part of the chosen system, ask;

"Is the root cause of this symptom a toxin? nutritional deficiency? parasite? or tissue damage?

Continue testing each choice until one tests strong. When you find the reason, the next step is to determine what particular toxin, parasite, tissue damage and/or nutritional deficiency, is causing the problem. If the reason is tissue damage, test which supplement will correct the tissue damage. If it is a toxin, parasite or nutritional deficiency, you will need to know specifically what it is.

Refer to the corresponding chart in the Appendix to determine the exact root cause, and select the perfect supplement to correct the imbalance naturally. If the root cause is toxins test, refer to the chart of toxins. If parasites test as the primary cause, refer to the chart of parasites, and the same with a nutritional deficiency.

To find the exact cause in any of the charts start by asking;

"Is the reason for this symptom on this chart? If yes, ask,

"Is it in the top half of the chart"

If the arm stays strong, the answer is true, and the reason is in the top of the chart. If the answer is weak, it is in the bottom half of the chart. This "shortcut" can save time. If the root cause is not on any chart, you have to test for the supplement that corrects the weakness, without knowing the cause.

Once you have concluded the cause is in either the top, or bottom half of the chart, name each toxin, parasite or nutrient on that half of the corresponding chart. As you test each of these choices ask;

"Is this the root cause of the problem?"

Name all the possibilities of toxins, parasites, or nutritional deficiencies, named on that half of the selected chart. One should test strong. That is your answer. You have now found the first reason for the health symptom. In the column with that particular toxin, parasite or nutritional deficiency is a supplement recommendation. These supplement choices, that I have used for years, are tried and true. There are other supplements on the market that will correct the problem, but I don't know what they are. Muscle testing gives you the freedom of choosing whatever supplement that you prefer. If it muscle tests that it will correct the situation, use it. It is not about what product is used. It is about results. Results speak loud and clear.

Remember, that once you have found the first reason, and corrected it, there can be another reason for the same symptom. There can be many reasons for the same symptom. To confirm that you have found all the causes of the symptom, ask;

"Is there another reason for this symptom?"

If there is another reason, start the process again by locating which system and repeat all the steps. Continue this process until there is no other reason for this particular symptom. Each symptom must be tested separately. The more precise you are in asking questions, the more accurate you will be, and you will get better results.

Muscle testing is great, because it is so precise, and accurate. Muscle testing is terrible, because it is so precise, and accurate. Always remember, if you make a general statement, or question, you will receive a general answer. This concept follows The Law of Attraction, what you focus on you receive. Ask more precise questions, you will receive deeper, more revealing, health secrets that your body is whispering. You now have the tool to do that.

THE TEN SYSTEMS OF THE BODY

In the next ten chapters, each system on the assessment form, is explained in detail. The most common health issues, of that particular system, are discussed. Questions and statements to use for muscle testing, for these symptoms, are included. This provides a good start on understanding how to use muscle testing to find real health problems. Once you learn the procedures, you can use the exact same questioning sequence to find any health issue in any system of the body.

The ten systems of the body are;

Circulatory: – blood, heart, arteries, veins, capillaries.

Digestive: - esophagus, lower esophageal valve, stomach, liver, gallbladder, bile ducts

Intestinal: small intestine – duodenum, jejunum, ileum. Colon

Glandular: adrenal, hypothalamus, pineal, pituitary, spleen, thymus, thyroid, parathyroid, ovaries, testicles.

Immune/Lymph: - GALT, WBC, Bone Marrow, Spleen, Thymus, Lymph fluid, lymph vessels, lymph nodes, cisterna chyli, thoracic/left lymph duct

Nervous: central nervous system, autonomic nervous system, cranial nerves, spinal nerves, nerve plexus, motor nerves, cutaneous nerves, sensory nerves

Reproductive: female and male reproductive

Respiratory: paranasal sinus, bronchioles, lungs

Structural: bones, joints, muscles, connective tissue, fascia, soft tissue

Urinary: kidneys, ureters, bladder, ureter

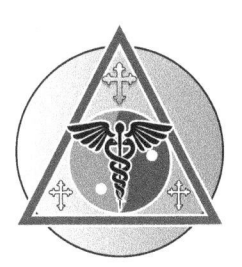

CHAPTER SIX

The Circulatory System – The Deliverer

In this chapter, you will learn the basic anatomy, and physiology of the circulatory system. This information corresponds with the choices which are on the Body Balance Healing System assessment form. The more you know about each system that you are testing, the more accurate your answers are, and the better the results will be.

Blood

Blood is the "river of life". It carries oxygen, and other nutrients, to every cell in the body, and brain. It helps eliminate waste from the cells. If blood is not flowing correctly, the body will suffer an imbalance in homeostasis, which eventually creates a disease.

Since blood flows to every cell of the body, the circulatory system is an important piece of the optimum health puzzle. . It is also the first choice on the assessment sheet. To test the blood, ask;

"Is the blood perfect?

If the answer is "no," ask;

"Is the blood viscosity perfect?"

If the test is weak, it is often the blood is too thick. Test the blood viscosity by asking;

"is the blood viscosity too thick?"

This can be caused by chronic dehydration, Vitamin E deficiency, excess fibrinogen and/or the liver. If the blood viscosity is too thick ask;

"Is it because of chronic dehydration? Vitamin E deficiency? excess fibrinogen? liver?"

Thick blood causes the heart to pump harder, causing high blood pressure. Find the reason why it is thick, and refer to the Appendix to correct the imbalance. Once that is corrected, ask again;

"Is the blood perfect?"

Repeat, and test the above causes to select the second reason in the blood. Always remember, there can be more than one reason for any symptom. Keep testing the same statement for the blood until there are no other reasons, and the blood is testing perfect.

The next question to ask about the circulatory system is;

"Is the blood flowing perfectly?"

If the blood viscosity is perfect, and the blood is not flowing perfectly, the cause is in one, or more of the choices provided on the assessment sheet. Ask;

"Is the reason for the lack of blood flow in the heart? arteries? arterioles? capillaries?"

This question can be asked more specifically, by adding the organ, gland, or tissue that you are testing.

"Is the blood flow perfect in the liver? spleen, kidneys?"

Once you have corrected the blood, ask;

"Is there anything else in the circulatory system causing this symptom?"

If the answer is "no," then move to the next system on the assessment sheet. If the answer is "yes," ask;

"Is the root cause in the heart? arteries? arterioles? capillaries? veins? venous capillaries?

If the question tests strong, you have discovered there is another reason in the circulatory system. Repeat the above procedures, find the part of the system that the problem is located. Ask;

"Is the root cause of this symptom a toxin, parasite, nutritional deficiency, or tissue damage?"

Heart

The heart is the next choice, in the circulatory system on the assessment sheet. Use the same questions as above, but substitute "heart," instead of "blood." The only difference in testing is the functioning number. All tissue in the heart should be functioning at 100% - not just sufficient (95%).

The heart is the pump for the arterial, venous and pulmonary blood flow. It contains its own electrical system. The natural "pacemaker" of the heart is the sinoatrial node. If you are experiencing racing heart, heart palpitations, fatigue, or high blood pressure, this is an area in our system that needs to be tested. The sinoatrial node is not on the basic health assessment. If your heart is the problem, and you are experiencing any of these symptoms, I would suggest testing the sinoatrial node.

"Is the sinoatrial node causing any of this symptom?"

The heart is so important it has its own blood vessels, called coronary arteries. The muscles in the heart are the cardiac muscles, and the nervous system is the cardiac conduction" system. To find the root cause in the heart ask;

"Is the root cause in the heart in the cardiac muscles? coronary arteries? cardiac conduction system?"

The heart has four valves – mitral, aortic, tricuspid and pulmonary valves. To determine whether any of the valves are causing any of the symptom ask;

"Is a heart valve causing any of these symptoms?"

Notice I specifically asked, "heart" valve. The reason I was specific is there are other valves in the body. Remember – the more specific your question, or statement is, the more accurate the answer will be.

Once you find the area of the heart where the root cause is, proceed with the exam, establishing the percentage of functioning and exact reason. Refer to the Appendix for supplements to correct it.

If you continue studying the Body Balance Healing System you will learn more about the heart.

Blood Vessels

The arteries are next in the circulatory system. These are the vessels that transport blood away from the heart. Clean blood is pumped out of the heart, and distributed through the aortic arch, to the entire body and brain. Anywhere that the arteries are not functioning perfectly creates a lack of blood flow, leading to nutritional deficiencies and eventually disease.

There are two separate blood flow systems that the heart supplies. These are the systemic and the pulmonary. Arteries are used in both. In the systemic circulation, the left ventricle of the heart pumps fresh blood through arteries, to all tissue in the body, and the brain. In the pulmonary circulation, arteries carry deoxygenated (dirty) blood from the right ventricle, away from the heart to the lungs

The veins do the exact opposite of arteries. Veins bring dirty, deoxygenated blood back to the heart through the inferior and superior vena cava into the right atrium of the heart. From there the blood is moved through the pulmonary arteries to the lungs. Once the blood is oxygenated, the veins move the blood back to the left atrium, through the left ventricle, where the life giving blood is pumped through the systemic arteries to the body, and the brain.

Both the arteries, and veins, have microscopic blood vessels. The arterial capillaries deliver oxygen, and nutrients to every tissue in the body. The smallest vessels of the veins are venous capillaries. They connect to the lymph vessels and assist in removing waste from the tissue.

Between the arteries and capillaries there are arterioles. These vessels are smaller than arteries, but larger than capillaries. They are the connection for blood flow from the arteries to the capillaries. Venules are part of the venule system that connect the veins, and venous capillaries.

In muscle testing, arterioles do not muscle test the same as arteries, or capillaries. Venules do not test as veins, or venous capillaries. To be more precise in your testing of the circulatory system, arterioles and venules should be included.

Once you determine that the root cause is in the blood vessels ask;

"Is the root cause in the arteries? arterioles? capillaries? veins? venules? venous capillaries?"

All of these can be weak when the veins initially muscle test weak. The same is true about the arteries. By asking about each of the three different sections of the artery, or vein, you will find the exact location. Remember, the more precise you are, the better your results will be.

Veins have a unique feature that arteries don't have. Vein valves are designed to keep blood flow from going back down, while the heart is trying to pump the blood from the feet, back to the heart. The heart can't pull blood from the feet, to the heart, in one beat. During the resting of the heart, without vein valves, the blood would follow gravity, pooling in the lower part of the legs. This is exactly what happens if vein valves are not working properly. Edema in the feet and ankles, sock lines, pain because of swelling in the lower leg area are all symptoms of vein valves not working sufficiently.

"Are all vein valves working sufficiently?"

The biggest concerns in circulatory are high blood pressure and heart disease. The medical field's answer to high blood pressure is prescribe a medication that will keep the numbers in range, but never fixes the root cause. Because the root cause is not being corrected, the symptom gets worse, and the second or third blood pressure pill is prescribed. The root cause of high blood pressure is never because of a deficiency of a drug.

To correctly muscle test blood pressure the systolic (top) and diastolic (bottom) have to be tested separately. These two numbers of your blood pressure represent two totally different actions of your heart – pumping and resting. To just test "blood pressure" is too broad of statement. It should be asked;

"Is the systolic blood pressure in range?"

"Is the diastolic blood pressure in range?"

If either test weak, find out the reason by asking;

"Is the reason in the circulatory system?"

If the answer is "yes," then muscle test the circulatory system, using the assessment sheet. If it is not caused by the circulatory system, test for the system where the root cause of the high blood pressure is located.

If you are suffering from fatigue, it could be caused by the circulatory system. The red blood cell (RBC) carries fresh oxygen to every tissue. This is called the oxygen carrying capacity. This refers to the ability of the RBC to do its job. When this is not working perfectly, the brain, and body do not receive sufficient oxygen. When the brain doesn't receive enough oxygen, fatigue, brain fog, and headaches are the symptoms.

"Is the oxygen carrying capacity working perfectly?"

If the answer is "no," asl;

"Is it because of B12?"

If "yes," ask;

"Can B12 be utilized on the red blood cell?"

The answer to this question tells the story. If it can be used on the red blood cell, the root cause is the shortage of intrinsic factor, secreted by the parietal cells in the stomach. This is caused by tissue damage of the parietal cell. Use Biotics Gastrazyme, which includes vitamin U. At the same time, sublingual B is a perfect choice to correct the oxygen carrying capacity while the parietal cells are being repaired. The sublingual B-12 is only a temporary fix while the real root cause is being corrected.

Once you have finished the natural health assessment for the circulatory system you have taken a big step toward getting healthier. Once it is corrected, you are insuring that your body, and brain, are receiving sufficient blood flow. The next system on the road to vibrant health is the digestive system.

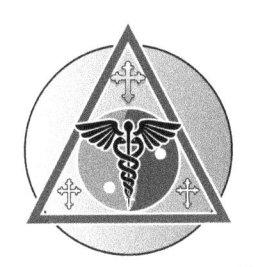

CHAPTER SEVEN

The Digestive System – the Food Processor

I remember a time I was teaching a class of 40 natural practitioners. I started my presentation by displaying my first power point slide – "You Are What You Eat." I asked, "how many of you believe this statement?" Over half the room of attendees raised their hands. I followed up with the next slide which shouted in big, bold, red letters "NO."

Yes, eating healthy is the first step to better health. Obtaining the cleanest organic foods is important, but what if you are not digesting those foods? You are only as healthy as the cell can utilize. Every cell in your body needs nutrition. If your body is not digesting your food properly, then it is impossible for the cells to receive the nutrients they need to continue functioning optimally. So, the secret of being healthy is not just what you eat, but what you digest and use. It is obvious if a person eats junk she/he cannot build a healthy body. But, eating healthy foods doesn't necessarily guarantee vibrant health and longevity.

There are four steps of utilization that have to work correctly in your body to be able to deliver the nutrients to your cells. In this chapter you will learn all of these steps in the digestion process to deliver the perfect nutrients to every cell in your body.

What is digestion? Digestion is the process of breaking down your foods so the nutrients from those foods can be absorbed into your body and eventually into the cell. Digestion is the breaking down of protein, fats, sugars, starches and fiber. If any of these are not being digested properly, the body will develop a deficiency of those nutrients, causing an imbalance in the body and over time, physical symptoms which create disease.

The first step in muscle testing how well your digestion is working is learning how to test protein digestion. The reason why protein digestion is so important is the body does not make protein nor does it store protein. Yet, there are nine essential amino acids that must be put into the body on a daily basis to create optimum health. These nine essential amino acids are found in complete protein. These eight essential amino acids then make up 22 different amino acids that configurate into thousands of different protein chains making all tissue in the body. This is why protein digestion is so important.

Patients visit me after they have already seen many outstanding doctors and well-known clinics. In many instances, through muscle testing, I discover the first major concern or imbalance is protein is not digesting properly. The sad thing is that when I ask them, "have any of these doctors told you that you are not digesting protein," the answer is always "no." None of these doctors checked one of the most important components of good health – digestion of protein and other nutrients.

Some of you who don't eat meat might think that you don't have to worry about your protein digestion. Please, don't make such a drastic mistake about your health. Almost all foods have some protein that must be digested properly. Whether you eat meat or not complete these three steps to make sure you are digesting protein.

The Digestive Process

Digestion is the breaking down of the foods we eat into smaller, usable substrates that the body uses at the cell level. If digestion is not functioning properly, it is impossible to get well. This is an imbalance that is affecting millions of people. The first system to test every time, whatever the symptom, is the digestive system. If you are not digesting your food, and your body is not using it, then whatever supplements or food is taken to correct the situation can't be utilized by the body. Let's start with making sure that all nutrients are being digested perfectly. We will start with protein.

Protein Digestion

The three steps to protein digestion;

1. Stomach digestion of protein
   This is the first step in the protein digestion cascade. HCl (hydrochloric acid) and pepsin are the two ingredients that mix together to start breaking down the protein into peptides. To muscle test to see if your protein is digesting perfectly ask;

"Is protein being digested perfectly?"

If the muscle test is strong (yes) proceed to the next nutrient – fat. If the muscle test responded weak (false) then you need to ask the following question to locate the exact cause. Ask;

"Is the reason why protein is not digesting perfectly hydrochloric acid Hcl or pepsin deficiency?"

If the question tests strong you have found your answer. Refer to the Appendix. If it tests false then ask the next question;

"Is a deficiency of protease causing this problem?"

Protease is an enzyme produced and secreted from the pancreas that completes the second step of protein digestion. If protease is the cause, refer to the Appendix and select the correct digestive enzyme by selecting the first choice of enzymes and asking;

"Now, by using this enzyme (speak the name of the enzyme product or place the bottle of enzymes against the subject's body) is protease perfect in protein digestion?"

If yes, you have found the enzyme that corrects the problem and is the one you should use at every meal. If no, continue testing the choice of enzymes until you find the correct enzymes to supply protease. Once this is found ask;

"Is protein now being digested perfectly/"

If the answer is yes (strong resistance) you are finished with testing protein digestion. If no, there are two enzymes that could be affecting the protein digestion – chymotrypsin and trypsin. Chymotrypsin and trypsin are produced in the pancreas and secreted into the small intestines through the common bile duct. Most digestive enzymes don't contain these two important enzymes for protein digestion. These two enzymes are the third step to complete the protein digestion process.

If one of these three areas is not working perfectly, digestion cannot possibly work. There can be more than one reason for these digestive system problems. That is why it is always important to ask the first question again after you find the first supplement. If after the testee holds the chosen supplement the muscle stays strong you have corrected the problem. If not, continue until protein is digesting perfectly.

What causes protein to not digest properly? The first step of protein digestion, which is controlled by the HCl and pepsin secretion, occurs in the stomach. Many people believe that HCl breaks down protein. But the truth of the matter is, it doesn't. HCl must combine with pepsinogen to create a very acidic liquid in the stomach called chyme. If either of these components is not correct then the first phase of protein digestion cannot be completed, and protein will not be digested properly. When this is the situation, a product that contains betaine HCl and pepsin should be recommended with every meal. It should be taken in the middle of the meal. But the most important thing if you forget is to get it in during that meal whenever you can. It is better late than never.

The Magic of Enzymes

Enzymes are crucial for digestion. Enzymes are catalysts which means they make things happen. They are able to break down foods. Enzymes are very specific. Protease enzymes break down protein. HCl is not an enzyme. Lipase enzymes break down lipids, which is the name for fats. Amylase enzymes break down starch. Disaccharide enzymes such as sucrase and maltase breakdown sugars. These are the types of enzymes which you need to understand to make sure your digestion is working perfectly.

There are two sources of digestive enzymes to help you get perfect digestion. The first source of enzymes is food enzymes. These are the enzymes that are in organic foods which are raw or steamed. Enzymes are very heat sensitive. Foods that are not organic or have been cooked over 118°F have had all of their enzymes destroyed. The second source of enzymes are supplemental digestive enzymes which supply the enzymes missing in the foods you are eating. This insures you are digesting your food properly every meal.

When you don't eat organic food or use a supplemental enzyme during your meal your body has to steal enzymes which normally would be used for other things in your body such as energy production. Think about the time after a Thanksgiving meal. When our whole family sits down for a dinner, I start by taking my enzymes, and passing the bottle of enzymes around the table for anybody else who would like to use some. What I have seen many times is the people who use enzymes at the meal have more energy after the meal and don't fall asleep watching TV. Why does this happen?

The liver produces digestive enzymes and metabolic enzymes, which are used for energy, tissue repair, and much more. If a digestive enzyme is not taken with every meal, the body robs "energy enzymes" from the liver to supply the digestive enzymes needed to digest the food that you just ate. Eventually this takes away valuable enzymes that are designed for other functions in the body. This enzyme depletion forces the body out of balance and creates symptoms and disease.

Fat Digestion

Fat digestion is a two-step process. The first step of digesting fats(lipids) is to emulsify the fats. This step is crucial for breaking down the grease on the fat before the enzymes can be effective. Think about emulsification like using detergent when you are washing dishes. You would not think about washing dishes in only water and expecting them to be clean. Emulsification is done by the bile which is produced by the liver and controlled by the gallbladder (if you have one). If you do not have a gallbladder it is imperative to use a supplement which includes bile with every meal.

After the stomach breaks down your food it travels out of the stomach into the upper part of the small intestines which is called the duodenum. Here is where the bile is transported from the gallbladder through the bile ducts into the upper part of the duodenum. This is timed perfectly by the body and is a crucial step for fat digestion. The second step to fat digestion is lipase which is produced and secreted by the pancreas through the pancreatic duct into the same area of the upper part of the duodenum. Both of these secretions must be perfect to digest fats.

"Are fats being digested perfectly?

If no, ask,

"Is fat being emulsified perfectly?

If no, add a bile digestive supplement (See Appendix)

When the fat isn't being digested perfectly, but emulsified perfectly, then the root cause is because of a lipase deficiency. Add a lipase digestive enzyme (See Appendix)

Carbohydrate Digestion

Carbohydrates are broken down into two different areas of digestion. The first one is starch. Starch digestion starts with salivary amylase, which is created by chewing your food. Salivary amylase is secreted by the salivary glands. This is the first step toward perfect digestion. The second step of digesting starch is pancreatic amylase, which is produced in the pancreas and secreted through the pancreatic duct into the duodenum.

"Is starch digesting perfectly?

If no, add a digestive enzyme that contains amylase. (See Appendix)

The second type of carbohydrate is sugar. Sugar is digested differently than starch although all starch eventually breaks down to sugar. Sugar digestion is controlled by the microvilli in the G.I. tract. These little fingers secrete disaccharides, which are different types of enzymes designed to break down the different types of sugars to usable glucose.

"Are all sugars digesting perfectly?

If no, add a digestive enzyme that contains disaccharide enzymes (See Appendix)

How can you tell if you are not digesting your food properly? The most obvious symptom is bloating, belching and/or burping. This is because of protein or sugar indigestion. When either one of these substrates isn't being digested properly, the undigested particles of food travel down into the lower G.I. tract. This undigested food starts fermenting and/or rotting causing gas and harmful bacteria. If you are not digesting fats, it can cause nausea, weight gain, hormone deficiencies and dry skin.

If you are having any of these symptoms the best advice is to start with two types of digestive aids. The first type should include betaine HCl (hydrochloric acid) and pepsin. This combination assists in digesting protein in the stomach by increasing hydrochloric acid. This supplement should be taken in the middle of the meal. Start with one and increase one capsule per meal until the stomach feels warm after taking the supplement. When this warmth is felt reduce by one supplement. That is the exact amount needed at this time but it can change. Any time the stomach feels warm after taking the supplement reduce again and again. Every time you reduce the supplement after the initial amount is a sure sign that your body's hydrochloric acid is improving.

The second digestive aid is a plant or pancreatic enzyme. On the label of a pancreatic or plant enzyme will be enzyme names such as sucrase, amylase, lipase, maltase, and many more. They all have one common, identifying mark- they all end in "ase."

There are two ways to use these plant enzymes. The first and most common is to take it during the meal to improve digestion. The second Is to help bloating and/or burping. When these symptoms appear, a protease enzyme taken without food (one hour before the meal or two hours after the meal) is needed. Taking enzymes on an empty stomach is a therapeutic technique, not digestive. The unused enzymes, not having to digest food, will travel down the G.I. tract and cleanup all of the undigested food particles which are causing the bloating and belching.

Muscle testing is so vital in balancing the digestive system. Millions of people suffer from digestive distress and the medical profession does not have the answer except for medication which never heals the root cause. With the ability to muscle test you don't have to guess what product you need. Your body knows what it needs and muscle testing is a simple and proven technique of communicating with the body's innate intelligence. In this chapter are muscle testing statements and questions which you can use that will help you get answers you're looking for to improve your digestion.

Anatomy of the Digestive System

Esophagus / Lower Esophageal Sphincter

Now that you know how to muscle test for digestion, the next areas to study are the various components of the digestive system, starting with the esophagus. If the root cause is in the esophagus use the basic procedures - establish the functioning number and reason(s) for the imbalance. Ask;

"Is the esophagus working sufficiently?"

If yes, go to the next choice. Ask;

"Is the lower esophageal sphincter working perfectly?"

The lower esophageal sphincter is a common problem for people. Notice that the question asked if the sphincter is working perfectly – not sufficiently. This valve, when working perfectly, shuts tight after food is moved from the esophagus into the upper part of the stomach. The lower esophageal sphincter is located at the bottom of the esophagus. When this valve is not working properly, it doesn't close tightly, which allows acidic contents to back up into the esophagus. This malfunction is the main reason for heartburn, gerd or acid reflux. These problems are not caused by too much hydrochloric acid (Hcl) as many medical doctors think. The question to ask is:

"Is the lower esophageal sphincter causing this symptom?"

If not move to your next choice; If yes, ask about each of the four main reasons that cause imbalance;

"Is it a toxin? nutritional deficiency? parasite? or tissue damage?"

When the reason is found refer to the Appendix for supplement recommendation

Stomach

When digestive problems occur, people initially think the issue is in the stomach. When the stomach muscle tests weak there are three areas which need to be tested.

The first section of the stomach is the cardia region. This is the upper part of the stomach where food arrives once the bolus (food) is moved down the esophagus. If you are suffering from nausea or stomach ache, this part of the stomach could be the culprit. This is a common breeding ground for H. pylori bacteria, especially if the HCl production is low.

"Is the cardia region of the stomach causing this symptom?"

If no, continue to the next choice. If yes, muscle test which of the four reasons is causing the malfunction and correct it as you did above.

The next area of the stomach is the body of the stomach. This is the section of the stomach where digestion happens. The HCl, pepsin, and gastric juices are secreted together. This acidic liquid is called chyme and begins the digestion process by breaking down amino acids and minerals.

"Is the body of the stomach causing this issue?" "Is the mucosa lining of the stomach causing this symptom?" "Is a deficiency of HCl the root cause?"

If yes, correct using the same process as above. If not, continue to the third area to test – the pyloric section. This includes the pyloric sphincter which is the valve that releases chyme (stomach gastric acid) into the next section of the digestive process – the small intestine.

"Is the pyloric sphincter causing this symptom?"

If the root cause is in the digestive system, but not in the stomach, the primary reason will be in one of the following areas.

The Liver

The liver is the largest and hardest working organ in your body. Your life depends on your liver. It is your main detoxifier and enzyme producer. It secretes bile, stores glycogen (available glucose), and has many other functions in the body. The main lobe of the liver is the right lobe. This is the largest part of the liver and located under your right rib cage. This lobe will be the most common section of the liver where you will discover your problem. There is also a left lobe of the liver, and some other smaller sections. At this level of teaching, the focus is on the right and left lobes of the liver.

Ask the question;

"Is the liver causing (the particular problem)?"

If the muscle test response is strong, or true, you have a choice – one is general, and the other is more specific. It is always your choice of how deep you want to test. This option pertains to any organ/gland where you find an imbalance. If you decide to do a general test, find the correct supplement that corrects the problem. Once the question "is the liver still causing this problem?" tests false, or weak, it is no longer the culprit. If you want to perform a more specific muscle test about the liver, start with the three primary detoxification phases. Here are questions to use;

"Is phase I in the liver working perfectly?"

"Is phase II in the liver working perfectly?"

"Is phase III in the liver working perfectly?"

All three of these phases are located in the right lobe of the liver. Phase I and phase II are the main two detoxifiers of the body. Their primary purpose is to keep toxins out of the blood. Phase III is involved in bile excretion.

If any of these phases are not working perfectly, they need to be corrected for optimum health. If Phase I or II aren't functioning one hundred percent, toxins are allowed to enter the bloodstream, and distributed throughout the body's tissue. This breach alerts the immune system, and creates inflammation. If Phase III is not perfect, the distribution of bile into the colon will affect the colon, and formation of the stool.

Gallbladder

This accessory organ of the digestive system is designed to be the storage compartment for bile, that is manufactured in the liver. Bile is the greenish fluid that helps digest fats (lipids). When the gallbladder is signaled by the intake of fat, it contracts, and forces the stored bile through the bile ducts, into the duodenum, where fats are emulsified.

The gallbladder gives many people problems. We have all heard the horror stories about gallbladder stones and attacks. The story closest to my heart is about our daughter – Leslie.

Late one Sunday night, Leslie's husband, Brian, called me, and told me that Leslie was in severe pain, and sitting in our local, hospital emergency room. He explained to me the pain was under her right ribcage. I remotely muscle tested her, confirming the root cause of the pain was her gallbladder. She had gallstones! I rushed to the hospital, and begged our daughter to come to our house. I warned her, if she stayed, they would do surgery. and remove her gallbladder before morning.

Although she was in severe pain, she did decide to come to the house. She walked up to the hospital receptionist, telling the lady she had changed her mind, and gave her the wristband. The receptionist, reacting in a surprised fashion, responded, "ok, honey, but you'll be back."

Leslie was in so much pain, she had to be gently lifted on to the massage table at our office, in our house. Michael, our son, also a Naturopath doctor, and I used electronics, natural supplements, and energy healing, which we call "white light" healing, for two hours. Once we finished, she raised herself off the massage table, and left the house with no pain. She has never had any pain since, and never had to go return to the hospital. Thank God for that healing.

With this story, I also want to add a caution. If you start getting symptoms of gallbladder imbalance, such as nausea, pain under the right rib cage that radiates into the back, or you have right shoulder pain, start now correcting the gallbladder. If you have sharp, persistent pain, you could possibly need emergency medical treatment. I hope you don't let it get that bad, but if it happens, please don't put off seeing a medical professional.

Many of the people who have had their gallbladders removed have problems digesting fats. When there is no gallbladder a digestive aid, with ox bile, at every meal is required.

Bile Ducts

Bile ducts are the tubes that move bile from the gallbladder, to the duodenum. When the gallbladder is removed, the bile travels straight from the liver to the duodenum constantly – not triggered, like the gallbladder. Often the bile ducts get adhesions, which is tissue sticking together and not allowing bile to flow properly.

"Are all bile ducts working sufficiently?"

If the answer is "no," ask;

"Is the problem in the bile ducts adhesions?"

Adhesions are caused by a lack of selenium, which is a trace mineral. In the Frequency Fingerprint program, explained later, the frequency for adhesions is 12.9-14.9 (twelve nine to the fourteen point nine power)

If you are muscle testing someone else, always confirm they still have their gallbladder, before you start testing their gallbladder. Nothing ruins your credibility as a reliable, muscle tester, faster than testing a gallbladder that is not there. You can either ask the person if they still have their gallbladder or muscle test by asking;

"Is the gallbladder present?"

If the arm stays strong it confirms there is a gallbladder, if it goes weak, the gallbladder has been removed.

Once you have completed the digestive system assessment, you know the root cause(s) of the digestive system's distress. Once you correct all the imbalances in the digestive process, ask the question;

"Is the digestive system still causing any of these symptoms?"

If the muscle test goes strong, the body is telling you there is at least one more reason in the digestive system, causing this particular symptom.

Repeat the above questions for the digestive system, as you again move through the choices.

Once the body responds weak to the above question, signaling there are no more reasons in the digestive system, move to the next step - utilization of the nutrients by your body.

Utilization of Nutrients

How well the cell receives a nutrient, and how effectively the body can use it as energy, and rebuilding, is utilization. Digestion is only the first of the four steps. The remaining three are, GI tract absorption, metabolism, and utilization at the cell level. Start by testing the next step – how well the nutrients are being absorbed.

1. GI tract absorption into the blood stream. Ask;

"Are all nutrients being absorbed through the GI tract into the blood stream sufficiently?"

If nutrients are not being absorbed properly, the GI tract receptors are the cause. Ask;

"Are all GI tract receptors working at least sufficiently?"

If they are not working at least sufficiently, it is usually a toxin. Confirm that it is a toxin through a muscle test, and then find the appropriate supplement, that will remove the toxin from the receptor. Once you have chosen the correct, supplement, place in against the body and ask;

"Are all GI tract receptors now working perfectly?"

If not, change supplements until you get a strong muscle response.

2. The liver must metabolize the nutrients perfectly. This takes place in the right lobe of the liver. Ask;

"Is the liver metabolizing all nutrients perfectly?"

If not, find the reason why it is not working perfectly, and add supplement(s) to correct the metabolism.

3. The last step is for the blood to deliver the nutrient to the cell. In the cell plasma membrane, there are "receptors" that work like the dish for our televisions. They lock in a particular nutrient, and bring it into the cell to be used. There are individual receptors for each nutrient. Ask,

"Are all nutrient receptors at the cell level working perfectly?"

Notice that with these three advanced questions, the correct answer will muscle test strong. By using these types of queries, a question that tests weak is an imbalance, which needs to be corrected.

If there are any problems in the utilization steps, correct them. If all answers stay strong, you are finished with digestion, and ready to move to the next system on the assessment sheet – the intestinal system.

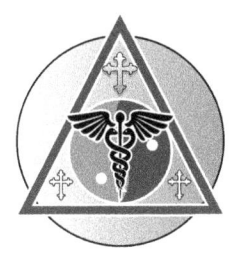

CHAPTER EIGHT

The Intestinal System – You Food Transporter

The saying goes, "You are only as healthy as your gut." As a digestive specialist, I agree with this popular statement. The question is," Why is that statement true?" Most patients who visit my office don't have a healthy gut. To get healthy, the first step is to work on correcting any problems in the GI tract (gastrointestinal tract). This chapter will discuss the intestinal system's anatomy, and physiology. It teaches how to muscle test the GI tract, and correct it naturally.

Think of the GI tract as a long tube. starting at the mouth, and ending at the anus. When I explain to patients that this tube is not actually *in* the body, they look shocked, but it's true. This inner tube is designed to digest, and absorb nutrients into the bloodstream. A nutrient is not actually "in" the body, until it reaches the bloodstream. If the GI tract is working properly, your food will be digested (broken down), and absorbed through the intestinal wall, into your bloodstream. The blood carries the nutrients into the tissue, and cells of your body. If it isn't working sufficiently, your body will suffer from malnutrition, no matter how well you eat.

The intestinal system is comprised of two distinct sections. The first section is the small intestine, which is comprised of three different compartments - the duodenum, the jejunum, and the ileum. Each of these areas is important for good digestion and absorption. If any of these sections are not working properly, your GI tract won't be functioning optimally, and your body will suffer.

The first part of the small intestines is the duodenum. It is connected to the lowest part of the stomach, which is the pyloric sphincter. This is the area of the small intestine that receive chyme, which is the acidic liquid from the stomach. There are two different sections of the duodenum.

The upper part of the duodenum is where many things are happening. The acidic liquid, chyme, from the stomach gets neutralized by bile from the gallbladder and/or liver that is released in this area. Chyme also gets neutralized by bicarbonate sodium from the pancreas that is secreted in this same area of the duodenum. If either one of these alkaline substances is not correct, the pH of the G.I. tract will be too acidic. Chyme is very acidic, like sulfuric acid. This acidic substance must be neutralized in this top half of the duodenum. If it does not get neutralized it will create inflammation in the gut and in severe cases this problem can cause ulcers.. Here are some questions to ask to test this area;

"Is the stomach acid being neutralized perfectly in the duodenum?"

If "no," ask;

"Is it because of a bile deficiency?"

If "no," go to next question. If "yes," find the root cause, and correct it by using the Appendix.

"Is it because of the gallbladder?"
"Is it because of the bile ducts?"

Ulcers are formed in the duodenum because of this acid dropping out of the stomach into this area. If you experience burning at the bottom of your sternum, it's a good possibility that you have ulcers in the duodenum. The reason this happens is a lack of a protective mucus, secreted by the Brunner's glands. These glands secrete mucus to protect the lining of the duodenum, so the acid from the stomach will not burn the tissue. The stomach acid is similar to sulfuric acid which would burn you if you touched it. As long as the Brunner's glands are protecting the tissue, the bile is being secreted perfectly, and the bicarbonate sodium is present then there should be no burning or problems in this area. If you are having these problems ask;

"Are the Brunner's glands working perfectly?"

"Are there any ulcers in the duodenum?"

"Is the bicarbonate perfect in the duodenum?"

If there are ulcers, refer to the Appendix for the correct supplement. If the bicarbonate sodium is not correct, refer to the glandular system, and test the pancreas, and pancreatic duct.

The duodenum is also the section of the small intestine where fats get emulsified. Bile, which is a detergent, degreases the fatty substances, so the lipase enzymes can digest the fats properly. If bile is not sufficient in the duodenum, the fat can't be emulsified nor digested perfectly. Ask;

"Are fats being emulsified perfectly?"

If "no," ask;

"Is the duodenum receiving bile perfectly?"

If "no," ask;

"Is this because of the gallbladder? liver? bile ducts?

Find the location of the root cause, then muscle test what is causing the imbalance

If fats are being emulsified, but not being digested perfectly, there is a deficiency of lipase - the enzyme that digests lipids (fats). The lipase enzyme is produced in the pancreas, and secreted through the pancreatic duct to the duodenum.

"Is lipase digesting fats perfectly?"

If the answer is "no," use a digestive enzyme that contains lipase, and refer to the pancreas section to locate the reason of the imbalance.

The second part of the duodenum should have more of an alkaline pH before it starts down the G.I. tract. If the pH is not corrected at this point in its journey down through the alimentary canal, there is no other place to correct it. This will create inflammation in the G.I. tract which can cause bloating, pain, leaky gut, and malabsorption. Ask;

"Is the pH perfect in the small intestine?"

If the answer is "no," the problem has to be either a bile, or bicarbonate deficiency. Refer to the above questions, and test again.

The second part of the small intestines is the jejunum. This is the main area where nutrients are absorbed. The wall of the jejunum is filled with finger looking projections called villi, which absorb nutrients, and micro-villi which secrete intestinal enzymes. Because of the folding of these villi, the amount of surface of nutrient absorption increases. If the villi are damaged, the body cannot absorb the required nutrients into the bloodstream. When this happens, the nutrients cannot be delivered to the cell. And remember, we are only as healthy as we are at the cell level. To test whether your nutrients are being absorbed properly ask;

"Are all nutrients being absorbed through the GI tract perfectly?"

If the answer is no, ask;

"Are all GI tract receptors working perfectly?"

There are receptors for each particular nutrient. If the receptor is not working perfectly than that nutrient will not be able to be absorbed. This is usually caused by a toxin. Ask;

"Are all Gi tract receptors free of all toxins?

If the answer is "no," refer to the toxicity chart, find the toxin, and remove it with the recommended supplement. Notice that these receptors are called GI tract receptors. There are other types of receptors in the body.

If the GI tract receptors are working perfectly, and nutrient absorption is still not sufficient, the villi is damaged. The reason for this damage of the villi is gluten. Say the word gluten real slow – g-l-u-e ten. Gluten sticks dough together, and it does the same thing to the micro-villi. Ask;

"Are the villi working perfectly? Are they free of tissue damage?"

"Are the micro-villi working perfectly?"

If either of these questions are false, refer to the Appendix for the correct supplement to repair the villi and/or micro-villi, and eliminate gluten from the diet.

Gluten is a protein, in wheat, that most humans have a difficult time digesting. Anybody who wants to be healthier needs to eliminate as much gluten from the diet as possible. It's not easy, because gluten is hidden in many foods, and condiments. This is another reason why muscle testing is so valuable. If you are concerned about eating gluten (and you should be), then muscle test the question;

"Is this food free of all gluten?"…all diary?…all preservatives…all sugars? …"

You can use muscle testing to test foods if they are organic. You can also muscle test for food allergies, by testing if there are any dairy, soy, preservatives, dyes, sugars, or anything you choose that you feel might be causing health problems. A good technique is hold the food you are wanting to test. While holding the substance, test whether the arm stays strong, or goes weak. No statement or question is needed. If the product is not good for your body, the arm will go weak.

Another part of the villi is the microvilli. The microvilli secrete disaccharide enzymes to digest sugar. If the microvilli are damaged, enzymes that digest sugars, called disaccharides, such as sucrase, maltase, and lactase are not secreted properly into the G.I. tract. When this happens, sugar is not digested properly. The symptoms of this issue are burping, belching, headaches, brain fog and lack of energy. Ask;

"Are the microvilli working perfectly?"

If not, refer to the Appendix for the appropriate supplement to correct the microvilli, and for the correct enzyme to use at every meal, while correcting the problem.

The reason for burping and belching is that when either protein, or sugars are not digesting properly. the undigested sugar/protein particles continue down the G.I. tract where they start fermenting. This fermentation causes gas, and excess of harmful, bacteria. The reason for headaches, brain fog, and lack of energy is a lack of glucose, caused by a sugar digestion issue. Sugar molecules are connected to the glucose molecule. If the disaccharide enzymes don't break down, and separate the sugar molecules, glucose can't be used as energy. If you are experiencing these symptoms ask;

"Is the GI tract free of all undigested sugar?"

If the muscle goes weak when testing for undigested sugar in the GI tract, use the appropriate enzyme for sugar digestion, and take it on an empty stomach (one hour before, or two hours after you eat). This can also be used for undigested protein. Ask;

"Is there any undigested protein in the GI tract?"

If there are undigested protein molecules in the GI tract, they will rot, causing gas and bloating. Use a protease enzyme on an empty stomach.

Many people suffer from a condition call dysbiosis, which causes inflammation and GI stress. It is caused by an imbalance of beneficial bacteria in the GI tract. This is usually caused by excess use of antibiotics, and medications. Remember, you can't be healthy without a healthy gut. To find out about the condition of the GI tract ask;

"Is my microbiome sufficient?"

Is my flora (beneficial bacteria) sufficient?"

"Is the balance of beneficial to non-beneficial bacteria sufficient?"

This is important to know because approximately 70% of the immune system is located in this special inner environment, where thousands of various bacteria co-exist. If there isn't sufficient "good" bacteria, then the "bad" bacteria takes control, and health starts to decline.

Probiotics will help, but the problem is that no probiotic on the market contains thousands of different species of bacteria in it's formula. I understand that the bottle claims it contains billions of bacteria, but it is billions of twenty or thirty types of bacteria. Experts estimate there is at least 300 – 1,000 species of bacteria. The only way to help the gut is to rebuild the environment, and allow the bacteria to naturally replicate and repopulate. This can be accomplished with fermented foods and supplements. A probiotic is always helpful, but attempting to replace all the microbiome with a probiotic is impossible. For more information refer to the Appendix.

Another major problem in the jejunum is leaky gut. Leaky gut is a situation where the junction cells of the jejunum, which are only one cell thick, get damaged. When this damage occurs, the junction cells, which are the cells that have the intelligence to know what should go into the blood, and what should be kept out, does not work properly. Think of a coffee filter in the older coffee makers. The reason a coffee filter was used was to keep the coffee grounds out of the coffee. But what if someone poked holes in the filter, what would happen? Of course, because of the bigger holes in the filter some of the grounds of the coffee would go into the brewed coffee. This is exactly what happens when someone has leaky gut. Increased intestinal permeability allows foreign substances into the bloodstream, which creates inflammation and autoimmune disease.

"Is the intestinal permeability perfect?"

If the answer is "no,", there are gut issues. When muscle testing the functioning of the intestinal permeability, when the functioning number muscle tests over 100%, there is leaky gut. use the recommended supplement from the Appendix.

"Is the intestinal permeability functioning over 100?"

When this question tests "yes," you have leaky gut.

The third part of the small intestines is the ileum. This lowest part of the small intestines is important, especially for the B12 absorption. To get absorbed, B12 has to couple with intrinsic factor, which is secreted from the parietal cells in the stomach. Without this absorption working properly, you will experience a lack of energy, because the B12 must be used in the hemoglobin of the red blood cell, to carry oxygen properly to your brain and body.

"Is the ileum working perfectly?"

"Is the IF-B12 complex being absorbed through the ileum perfectly?"

If not, refer to the Appendix. If B12 is not being absorbed properly, use a sublingual B12. If B12 is not being absorbed, it is due to tissue damage in the parietal cells of the stomach. To confirm this, ask;

"Is the intrinsic factor being made perfectly."

If not, the parietal cells, in the stomach, need repaired. Refer to the Appendix.

There is a valve at the end of the small intestine called the ileocecal valve. This valve keeps the liquid that is now entering the colon from backing up into the small intestines. This valve can be stuck open or stuck closed. Either way it will give you health challenges. Ask;

"Is the ileocecal valve working perfectly?"

If not refer to the Appendix and then find the one that will make that question true (strong).

The Large Intestine (Colon)

The second part of the intestinal system is the colon, large intestine or bowel. Known best for elimination of waste, the colon does so much more. Some nutrients are manufactured in the bowel by beneficial bacteria. The ascending colon reabsorbs water back into the body. If you are experiencing diarrhea, constipation, or flatulence ask,

"Is the colon causing this symptom?"

If the answer is "yes," ask;

"Are all nutrients being made sufficiently in the colon?"

"Is the ascending colon reabsorbing water perfectly?"

"Is the colon sufficient in beneficial bacteria?"

If any of these questions test weak, then do as directed in the Appendix.

The colon has six sections – Caecum, ascending colon, transverse colon, descending colon, sigmoid colon and rectum. All six sections must work sufficiently (at least at 95%) to have a healthy bowel elimination.

Peristalsis is the movement of the fecal matter through each of these sections. This is performed by the taenia coli, and smooth muscles, that travel through all six sections of the colon. Each section of the colon has its own set of smooth and circular muscles. Different parts of taenia coli ribbon through each area. All colon activity, like the entire GI tract, is governed by the enteric nervous system, which is part of the autonomic nervous system.

If a person is experiencing symptoms of constipation, diarrhea, flatulence, or cramping test the peristalsis by asking;

"Is the peristalsis functioning at least sufficiently?"

If peristalsis is not working sufficiently, refer to the Appendix.

Constipation is another big problem for Americans. Laxatives are one of the most popular over-the-counter purchases. Why? Because Americans don't like to think, or talk about poop. Yet, Dr. Bernard Jensen, a well-respected pioneer in natural health, quoted, "all illness starts in the bowel."

While the cause of diarrhea is usually in the small intestine, constipation is usually a colon problem. Although, it can be other areas such as the thyroid. Nothing feels worse than a backed-up colon. Many people rely on laxatives, which over time destroy the muscle tone in the colon, guaranteeing a lifetime dependency on laxatives.

The big question I hear the most is; "what is a normal bowel movement?" The answer depends on who you ask. Medical doctors claim that one bowel movement per week or day is fine. All natural health practitioners will strongly disagree. The perfect number of bowel movements per day is the number of meals you consume per day. One or two bowel movements per day is good for most of us.

Some of the reasons for constipation are stress, a nutritional deficiency, lack of fiber, insufficient water intake and/or lack of exercise. Also, underactive thyroid activity (hypothyroid) will cause this problem. If the body tests that it is experiencing constipation, muscle test each of these reasons, and see if any of them are causing constipation. Ask;

"Is _____ causing constipation?"

If the answer is "yes," to any of these reasons, refer to the Appendix. Choose each supplement suggested, starting with the first choice, have the person being tested hold the supplement against their body, and then ask the question again. Some of these reasons can be corrected by supplements, and some can't be resolved in that manner. Lifestyle changes such as improved diet, meditation, exercise, and more water are needed. A good way to use muscle testing to know what is actually causing the problem or helping it is ask;

"Is this food (or supplement) causing constipation (or diarrhea)?

"Will this food (or supplement) improve the constipation (or diarrhea)?"

Another colon problem Americans experience is flatulence – the proper name for gas escaping the anus. This gas is proof that there are issues in the colon. In most cases it is caused by rotting protein. Undigested, or under-utilized protein, accumulates in the colon where it rots, producing not only gas, but harmful bacteria. When the undigested food is protein it is called indican, which is usually the main reason for the flatulence.

"Is the colon free of indican?"

If "no," refer to the Appendix to learn about probiotics for the bowel.

Another reason for gas in the bowel is food is moving through too slow. To muscle test for the answer ask;

"Is the motility of the colon working perfectly?"

Often a lack of water, fiber, magnesium, or Vitamin C is causing the constipation. Test each of these separately by asking;

"Is _____ (put in which ever nutrient you are testing) causing any of this constipation?"

If "yes," refer to the suggestions for that particular nutrient.

Sometimes the primary "root cause" for constipation is not in the colon. Nerve innervation (nerve supply) to the taeniae coli, and other areas of the colon is not working sufficiently. This is controlled by the enteric nervous system. A lack of nerve energy will slow the movement of the colon. To find out ask;

"Is all muscles and teniae coli receiving sufficient innervation or nerve supply?"

If the answer is "no," ask;

"Is this because of the enteric nervous system?"

If "yes," correct the imbalance. If the root cause of this problem is not in the enteric nervous system, but it is in the nervous system, refer to the nervous system assessment.

The colon is one of the major elimination systems of the body. If the colon is not working properly, the body will turn toxic. Waste will recycle into the blood stream, and tissue. This creates an acidic body, which turns into disease. By making sure your colon is eliminating sufficiently is a big step toward optimum health.

This concludes this chapter on the intestinal system. Refer to this chapter when your GI tract is showing signs of distress. There is more to learn about the intestinal system, but this information will help you get started solving many of your gut issues.

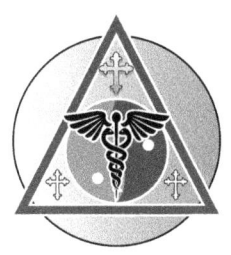

CHAPTER NINE

The Glandular (Endocrine) System – Your Hormone Supplier

Hormones are the messengers of the body. The glandular, or endocrine system is a group of glands, which produce, and secrete different hormones. Each hormone communicates with a particular group of cells in the body. In this chapter, each gland that is included on the natural health assessment, is addressed. The glands are in alphabetical order, so it is easier to locate the gland you are wanting to test. The first set of glands are the adrenal glands.

The Adrenal Glands

The adrenal or renal glands sit on top of the kidneys. They are the major "stress" related glands. Adrenal exhaustion has become a normal in this hectic crazy world. If you, or the person being tested, is suffering fatigue there is probably an imbalance in the adrenals. The adrenals are connected to the thyroid, and both are the backup for the heart. This makes them important glands to balance when having these symptoms.

The adrenals have two main sections – adrenal medulla and adrenal cortex. The adrenal medulla produces norepinephrine and epinephrine (adrenalin). This area of the adrenals produce extra adrenaline when a person is experiencing fear – real or imagined. The person experiences the 3 F's – fight, flee or freeze. When fear is perceived, the sympathetic nervous system triggers the adrenals to produce excess adrenalin. This over active production continues until the threat is gone. This survival mechanism was designed to perform at this maximum output for a short period of time. But, living in stress, day after day, the adrenals get worn out. At that time, the person suffers adrenal exhaustion, which causes severe fatigue, anxiety, nervousness, sleep issues, and high blood pressure.

If there is anxiety, nervousness, not being able to sleep, the adrenal medullas are over active. If you are suffering from fatigue and exhaustion, the adrenal cortex is under active. Muscle testing will tell you how the adrenals are functioning. Start by asking;

"Are the adrenals causing any of these symptoms?"

If the answer is "yes," test each section to locate the exact area in the adrenals.

"Are the adrenal medullas causing any of these symptoms?"

When the adrenal medulla muscle tests strong to that question, the functioning can be under active or over active. You will need to test for the functioning to decipher whether the tissue involved is over or underactive . Don't assume. Always test.

"Are the adrenal medullas over-active?

This one question will give you the answer. If the answer is "no," the adrenal medulla is under-active. If the answer is "yes," muscle test for the root cause and correct it. The next question is;

"Is the root cause of why the adrenals are (either over-active or over-active) in the adrenal medulla?"

If the root cause is in the adrenal medulla, correct the problem, but if the root cause is not in the adrenals, test the HPA axis, which is discussed later in this chapter.

The adrenal cortex has three separate "zonas". The first zona is the Zona Reticularis, which is responsible for DHEA, pregnenolone, progesterone, estrogens and testosterone. The Zona Fasciculata secretes cortisol. The third zona is the Zona Glomerulosa, which controls aldosterone. To test if these areas are functioning sufficiently ask;

"Are all zonas of the adrenal cortex functioning sufficiently?"

If "no," ask;

"Is the Zona Reticularis working sufficiently? Zona Fasciculata? Zona Glomerulus?"

Start by correcting the adrenal cortex as a whole. Once muscle testing confirms that the adrenal cortex is functioning at least sufficiently, test each of the separate zonas to make absolutely sure there are no other problems. Testing each zona is a more specific test, which will deliver a more precise answer and better result.

The Hypothalamus

The hypothalamus is the "control tower" of the body. Located in the limbic center of the brain, it regulates the autonomic nervous system of the body. The HPA axis – the hypothalamus, pituitary and adrenals together, supply the hormones for the adrenals, thyroid and gonads.

If you, or the person being tested, experience hormone deficiency symptoms such as hot flashes, low libido, fatigue, hair loss, and/or irritability, you can find where the problem is located by muscle testing the following questions;

"Is the hypothalamus producing hormones sufficiently?"

"Is the anterior pituitary gland secreting hormones sufficiently?

"Is the HPA axis working sufficiently?"

If the HPA axis is not working sufficiently, separately test;

Is the hypothalamus functioning at least sufficiently? the anterior pituitary? The adrenal?

If the HPA axis is not functioning at least sufficiently, one or more of these glands is out-of-balance.

The Pancreas

The pancreas is the next gland on the natural assessment. The three functions of the pancreas are insulin, digestive enzyme and sodium bicarbonate production. Insulin production happens in the beta cells, in the Isle of Langerhans. The pancreas secretes pancreatic enzymes – lipase, protease and amylase. It also produces sodium bicarbonate. To evaluate the functioning of the pancreas, ask;

"Is the pancreas producing insulin sufficiently?"

If the pancreas is not producing sufficient insulin, there will be excess glucose in the blood. When this imbalance becomes more severe the person suffers from diabetes.

"Is the pancreas producing sodium bicarbonate perfectly?"

Sodium bicarbonate neutralizes the acidic chyme, dripping out of the stomach, into the upper part of the duodenum. Without sodium bicarbonate, the excess acid would make the pH of the GI tract too acidic, which would cause many gastric problems.

"Is the pancreas producing all digestive enzymes sufficiently?"

If the pancreas is not producing enzymes sufficiently, start by finding the correct enzyme to take at every meal, until the imbalance has been corrected. Test the pancreas enzyme production, find the root cause of the problem, and correct it. If food is not being digested properly because of a deficiency of a pancreatic enzyme, but the enzymes are being produced sufficiently by the pancreas, the pancreatic duct should be tested;

"Is the pancreatic duct working sufficiently?"

"Is the duodenum receiving all digestive enzymes, sodium bicarbonate, and bile sufficiently?"

If "no," refer to the Appendix for the best supplement to correct the pancreas or pancreatic duct.

The Pineal Gland

The pineal gland is the next gland on the natural health assessment. Although this gland is not involved as much as other glands, it is important to the body's health. The pineal gland is the gland of the third eye. It is known as "the light keeper." The main function is the production of melatonin. Melatonin is the main hormone that controls sleep. If there are sleep issues, the pineal gland could be the problem. Ask;

"Is the pineal gland producing melatonin sufficiently?"

If "no," refer to the Appendix, and get the perfect product to correct the pineal gland.

The Pituitary Gland

The pituitary gland is referred to as the "master "gland because it controls the output of hormones to most of the major glands. It produces antidiuretic hormone, ACTH (Adrenocorticotropic hormone), TSH (Thyroid-stimulating hormone), FSH (Follicle-stimulating hormone), and LH (luteinizing hormone).

When there is a health issue in the thyroid, adrenals, or gonads, the primary cause is not always in the gland where the symptom seems to be. Find out by muscle testing if the root cause is in the gland that is not functioning sufficiently. If the root cause is not in the target gland, the root cause could be in the pituitary gland, or the hypothalamus. If the hypothalamus is not producing, and/or secreting the correct amount of releasing hormones to the pituitary, then the pituitary can't secrete the correct hormones to the other glands.

Once it is confirmed that the problem is in the glandular system, start your search for the root cause of the first symptom by asking;

"Is the root cause of this problem in the glandular system?"

Never assume the root cause is where the problem exists, or even in the same system. If the muscle test discovers that the root cause is not in the glandular system, test each system to find the system where the root cause is located.

If muscle testing confirms that it is in the glandular system, then continue through the glandular system by asking;

"Is the root cause in the thyroid? Adrenals? Ovaries? Testes?"

If none of these tests true, then move to the next step up the chain of the HPA Axis;

"Is the root cause in the pituitary?"

If the root cause is in the pituitary, refer to the Appendix to correct it. If it is not in the pituitary, then ask;

"Is the root cause in the hypothalamus?"

When there is a problem in the glandular system you can also start from the top and move down. The hypothalamus can be tested first, then the anterior pituitary, and the adrenals, thyroid and/ ovaries or testis. Either way, muscle testing will show you where the root cause is located, and how to correct it naturally.

The Thyroid Gland

The thyroid gland is located in the neck. It produces thyroxin hormones- T1,T2,T3, and T4, which control metabolism and heat production. If the thyroid is underactive (hypothyroid), the body will be cold and sluggish. Weight issues and hair loss are two other effects of an underactive thyroid. When the thyroid is underactive the TSH (thyroid stimulating hormone) level in the blood will be high, indicating that the thyroid is underactive. This factor is not true all the time. If your thyroid is not functioning perfectly ask;

"Is the primary (root cause) reason for the thyroid not functioning perfectly in the thyroid?"

If "yes," find the function, and cause, then refer to the Appendix. If not, ask;

"Is the reason the thyroid is not functioning sufficiently because of the pituitary?" If no, ask;

"Is the hypothalamus causing the thyroid to not function perfectly?"

In most cases, the root cause will be in one, or more of these glands. Refer to the hormonal cascade for thyroid hormones. The cascade starts with the hypothalamus providing different "releasing hormones." These releasing hormones are used by the pituitary, and then re-released as hormones to the thyroid, adrenals and gonads.

The Thymus Gland

This almost forgotten gland, which people mistakenly believe is not important because it shrinks as we age, is an intricate part of the glandular system by producing thymosin, which stimulate T-Cell development. Optimum T-cells are crucial in the immune and lymph systems.

The thymus gland is located in the middle of the chest, behind the sternum. It is the place that Tarzan pounded his chest. By humming while tapping the sternum area, you will be able to find the exact spot. The "perfect" place will produce a vibration you will know is right.

The thymus gland is also used to correct polarity. Donna Eden introduced the "thymus thump," which we still use today, to correct polarity. By tapping on this area with your fingertips, or loose fist, as you breath deep slow breaths, polarity will be corrected. This thymus tapping is good to start the day, or anytime you feel tired or stressed. It strengthens the immune system, re-energizes the body, and improves the lymph system.

The Parathyroid Gland

There are two small glands located on each side of the thyroid. These four glands are the parathyroid glands. Their main function is to regulate calcium in the blood. Always working to keep the blood perfect in calcium, the parathyroid can excrete calcium if there is excess, or can rob calcium from the bones if the serum level decreases. Either a low parathyroid or hyper parathyroid will throw calcium levels off.

Too much calcium will result in arteriosclerosis, kidney stones and calcium deposits which cause bone spurs. A deficiency of calcium creates a more acidic pH for the body, which translates to pain and disease. It also causes osteoporosis.

"Is the parathyroid gland working perfectly?"

"Is calcium perfect in the blood?"

If this gland, or any other gland, is not functioning at least sufficiently, find out if the root cause is in that particular gland. If it tests that the root cause is in the tissue of that gland, refer to the Appendix for the supplement to use to correct the problem. If the root cause is not in the affected gland, find the root cause and correct it. By correcting the root cause will correct the gland it is affecting.

Hormones are an important component of abundant health. All hormones are produced by a particular gland. There are many hormones in the body besides the ones discussed in this chapter. Every hormone is important, and a deficiency of one hormone can cause an imbalance in the body. Correcting these "major" glands and hormones is a positive approach toward balancing the body. The glands in this chapter are involved in many common health complaints. Learning how to muscle test for deficiencies in these glands will guarantee a better, more vibrant life!

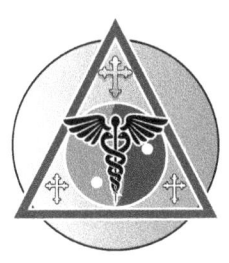

CHAPTER TEN

Immune/Lymphatic System – The Protector

The immune, and lymphatic systems work hand in hand, cleansing the body of waste, and protecting the body. If either one is not working properly, the other is also being negatively affected. If you suffer from allergies, get sick frequently, can't get well, or have edema, you are showing symptoms, indicating that these two systems are not working sufficiently.

The immune system is comprised of the bone marrow, GALT, spleen, lymph system and thymus gland.

The Bone Marrow

The bone marrow is a major contributor to the immune system by supplying the white blood cells. The white blood cells are the army, and protectors of the blood and body. When WBC count is low, the body will not be able to defend itself. To determine white blood count, muscle test;

"Is the white blood count perfect in the blood?"

If WBC are not perfect in the blood, it must be determined whether they are too low, or too high. Ask;

"Are there more white blood cells in the blood than normal?"

A "yes," answer denotes an infection in the body, and the army of white blood cells are hard at work, fighting off an enemy. To find the root cause of the elevated white blood cell count, refer to the chapter on parasites.

"Are the white blood cells less than normal?"

If that is true, ask:

"Is the root cause of the low WBC in the bone marrow? thymus gland? "

A blood test that shows an elevated white blood cell count signals an infectious agent (parasite) present in the body. To find the parasitic source causing the increased WBC count, test each system by asking;

"Is the reason for an elevated WBC count in this system?"

Continue testing until a system tests true. Test through that system to find the exact location, and cause. Correct that cause, and then repeat the test to make sure there are no more sources.

The Galt

The largest part of the immune function is the GALT (gut-associated lymphoid tissue). This comprises approximately 70% of the immune function. The GALT is interconnected to the microbiome in the gut. This environment of thousands of types of bacteria directly communicate with the brain, via the brain-gut connection.

If antibiotics or medications have been used, a rebuilding of the inner terrain is a must. Probiotics are a good step in the right direction, but not enough. The GALT has beneficial bacteria, that still hasn't been discovered. The best probiotic has less than one hundred different strains. Instead of trying to replace the strains of bacteria, is to rebuild the inner terrain of the gut with fermented foods, probiotics, and prebiotics. This imbalance can be found and rebuilt by asking;

"Is the GALT working perfectly?"

If the answer is "no," ask;

"Will a probiotic repair the damage?"

If it answers "yes," start on a probiotic immediately. If "no" refer to the Appendix for recommendations of a supplement that will regrow the inner terrain, and repopulate the bacteria of your microbiome.

"Is the GALT functioning perfectly?"

"Is the microbiome perfect?"

"Is the brain-gut connection working perfectly?"

"Is the gut - brain working perfectly?"

If any of these questions tests weak, refer to the Appendix for recommendations.

The Spleen

The spleen is the main organ of the immune, and lymph system. The white pulp of the spleen is dedicated to the immune system. Michael, our son and also a Naturopath doctor, explains the spleen perfectly. "The spleen is the mucus queen." If you are suffering from excess mucus in your throat, or respiratory areas, don't rule out problems in the spleen.

The spleen controls many of the immune functions for other organs and glands. Because the spleen also helps clean blood, toxins can lodge in spleen tissue, causing immune function to weaken. This diminishes the body's ability to resist disease.

The Thymus Gland

The thymus gland is located in the middle of the chest, where Tarzan pounded his chest. Donna Eden made it famous with the "thymus thump". The thymus gland is not only a gland, but also an important component of the immune system. It matures white blood cells. The thymus gland is frequently overlooked, but it should not be forgotten. If the bone marrow makes perfect white blood cells, but the thymus does not mature them, the immune system suffers.

The thymus gland is used to correct polarity. "Polarity" is the ability of the body to respond in a true fashion when muscle tested. If you, or the person being tested, is not in polarity, true will test false and false will test true. Use the thymus thump, while deep breathing to correct polarity. It only takes a minute, and well worth the time, and effort, if you are feeling tired, stressed, or out of polarity. It's a great idea to start every morning doing thymus tapping.

Here are some questions for your spleen and thymus. Ask;

"Is the white pulp of the spleen working sufficiently?"

"Is the thymus working or functioning perfectly?"

If either one is not functioning at least sufficiently, your immune system and lymphatic system are compromised. Follow the basic protocols to find the reason why that area is not functioning at least sufficiently. Refer to the Appendix.

The Lymph System

The lymph system is a combination of glands or nodes, ducts, and vessels. There are more lymph vessels than circulatory vessels in the body. The lymph's main function is to eliminate waste from the tissue. If this is not working properly the waste starts backing up in the tissue. This causes acidosis, inflammation and pain. To test the lymph system, start with the lymph fluid. Ask,

"Is the lymph fluid's viscosity perfect?"

Viscosity means thickness. You want the viscosity of the lymph perfect so it will flow throughout the lymph system. If it is too thick, the lymph system is will struggle to eliminate the waste from the body. If the lymph fluid is too thick, it is often because the liver is not detoxing toxins properly, and is dumping the excess into the lymph fluid. If this is happening, muscle test the liver to determine if it is detoxing toxins perfectly.

"Is the liver causing the lymph fluid to be too thick?"

If the answer is "yes," then muscle test the right lobe of the liver for the root cause. If the answer is "no," then test the lymph fluid and correct it.

Lymph Glands/Lymph Nodes

The lymph glands or lymph nodes are the filter centers for the lymph waste. These groups of glands are situated throughout the body. The main collections are in the neck, groin and armpits. The "micro lymph system" includes the afferent lymph vessels and the lymph capillaries. These microscopic vessels carry waste from the tissue and cells and transport it to the lymph nodes. Lymph nodes filter the waste, and move it to the efferent lymph vessels, which move the waste from the lymph node to the macro lymph, which dumps into the subclavian vein.

If you are feeling swollen glands or lymph nodes ask;

"Is the micro lymph system causing this symptom?"

If the answer is "Yes," ask;

"Are all lymph glands or lymph nodes working at least sufficiently?"

"Are all lymph capillaries working at least sufficiently?"

"Are all afferent lymph vessels working at least sufficiently?"

"Are all efferent lymph vessels working at least sufficiently?"

If the answer is "no," then the answer is in the macro lymph system, which includes the thoracic duct or left lymphatic duct and the cisterna chyli. To find the root cause ask; "Is the cisterna chili causing this symptom?" thoracic duct? left lymphatic duct?"

The lymph system doesn't have a pump, like the circulatory system. The lymph is moved by muscle. The two ways to move lymph are through movement, and deep breathing. The best exercise to move lymph is by jumping up and down. Vertical movement is the best to move the lymph, but any exercise helps.

Deep breathing is a wonderful way to move the lymph fluid. Start the deep breathing by focusing your inhalation of breath in your pelvic region. Continue deep breathing as you imagine moving the air to the top of your head.

A breathing exercise that I teach is called the 1-4-2 method. While filling your lungs with air count to five or whatever your number is comfortable to you. Next, hold your breath for a count that is four times the seconds you inhaled. Exhale through your mouth, as if you are blowing out a candle. Exhale twice the time you inhaled, or half the counts you held your breath. For instance, if you counted to five as you inhaled, you would hold your breath for a count of twenty. Then you would exhale for a count of ten. The last exit of air that you force out allows the lymphatic system to move.

Think of it as a ratio of 1 – 4 – 2. You can start at any amount of inhaled counts. Don't judge yourself if you can't do five or three. Start wherever you are comfortable, and keep doing it. You will improve and get stronger. As an example, if you inhaled for a count of 3 you would hold your breath a total count of 12 and exhale for a count of 6. If you had a beginning inhalation of 5 you would hold a count of 20 and exhale for a count of 10.

CAUTION: Be careful when doing the breathing exercise. If you have respiratory issues or any other health condition that might cause you harm, either don't do the exercise, or start at a lower number and build your way up.

Lymphatic Ducts

There are two lymph ducts. The right lymphatic duct drains waste from the upper right quadrate of the body. The thoracic or left lymphatic duct drains the rest of the body. All lymphatic flow dumps into these two ducts, which are connected to the venous system.

If you have lymph nodes swelling on only one side of your body, muscle test the lymphatic duct of that specific side. Many times you will discover it is not functioning sufficiently.

"Is the thoracic or left lymphatic duct working at least sufficiently?"

"Is the right lymphatic duct working at least sufficiently?"

"Is the lymph system able to drain into the blood at least sufficiently?"

If the answer to this last question is "no", muscle test which part of the lymphatic system is not working at least sufficiently. The root problem might not be in the lymph system. If the root cause is not in the lymph system, the problem could be in the blood or the kidneys. If the kidneys are not filtering blood perfectly, there will be toxins in the blood. When the blood is full of toxins, the lymph system will not be able to dump toxins into the blood.

"Are the kidneys filtering all toxins perfectly?"

"Is the lymph system able to drain into the blood?"

Remember if there are toxins in the blood, either the nephrons in the kidneys or the detoxification pathways in the right lobe of the liver are not functioning perfectly.

This is the end of the immune/lymph system section. It is the fifth of the body systems. You have finished half of the ten systems of the Body Balance Healing System. One suggestion to make your testing faster is to ask;

"Is the root cause of this problem in the top (first half) of the assessment sheet?"

If the answer is "no," the root cause is in the bottom half of the assessment sheet, and you don't have to muscle test the top five systems. If the answer is "yes," you don't have to be concerned about the bottom half of the systems. This is definitely a time saver.

You are now ready to move to the second half of the assessment sheet. The sixth system is the nervous system.

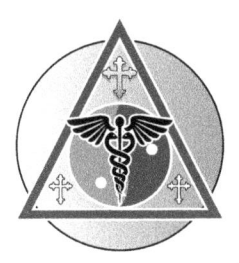

CHAPTER ELEVEN

The Nervous System – Your Information Carrier

The nervous system is the electrical system of the body. This electrical energy is information. It is carried through a vast network of nerves, and neurons, throughout the body and the brain, communicating with every cell. All five senses are constantly monitoring stimuli from the environment. The stimuli are carried from the sensory receptors, through the sensory nerves, to the brain. The brain receives the message, translates it into directives, and sends them to the appropriate part of the body. If it were not for the nervous system, the body could not detect physical pain or move a muscle. The heart wouldn't beat, and the brain couldn't think.

Brain/Spinal Cord

The central nervous system (CNS) is the first choice on the assessment sheet. This consists of the brain, and spinal cord. When the root cause is in the central nervous system decide which area it is located by asking;

"Is the root cause of this problem in the brain?"

The cerebral cortex is the covering of the brain. It consists of five lobes – frontal, limbic, occipital, temporal and parietal. To find the root cause in the brain ask;

"Is the root cause in the cerebral cortex?"

If "yes," then test each section of the cerebral cortex.

"Is the root or primary cause in the frontal lobe? limbic system? occipital? parietal? or temporal lobe?"

Find and measure the functioning of the tissue causing the problem. Once you determine the functioning percentage, test for the cause of the problem. Ask;

"Is it a toxin? Parasite? Nutritional deficiency? Tissue damage?

Advanced muscle testers can use the exclusive "Fingerprint Frequency" program discussed later in the book. Once you have found the cause, refer to the corresponding chart in the Appendix for the correct supplement.

If the body responds "no" through muscle testing, then the root cause of this particular problem is in the spinal cord. To double check the accuracy of the testing ask;

"Is the root cause in the spinal cord?"

If the first test confirmed that the root cause was in the nervous system, and in the central nervous system, and isn't in the brain, it has to be in the spinal cord. Use the same procedure – find the functioning, the cause and rebalance the tissue.

Cranial Nerves

Cranial nerves are another integral part of the nervous system. These nerves of the brain are the pathways for all the information from the senses to be received and transmitted to the body. The largest cranial nerve is the vagus nerve. The name "vagus" means "wandering." True to its name, the vagus nerve travels from the medulla oblongata, by the esophagus, and wanders throughout the GI tract, liver and intestine to the bowels and bladder.

The vagus nerve controls peristalsis, or motility, of the digestive system, from the esophagus to the colon. Motility is the continuous movement of food particles, moving through the GI tract. This is accomplished by smooth muscles, which are controlled by part of the vagus nerve called the enteric nervous system.

"Are all cranial nerves working sufficiently?"

"Is the vagus nerve working sufficiently?"

"Is the enteric nervous system working sufficiently?"

In some questions or statements "sufficiently" is acceptable, because if tissue is functioning sufficiently (at least 95%), that tissue won't cause any symptoms. In certain areas of the body such as the liver, brain and heart, the tissue should be working perfectly. Of course, in all instances working perfectly (100%) is always the best. In most cases the body doesn't react until the tissue is functioning under 95% (not sufficient) except for the areas just mentioned.

The Spinal Nerves

The next part of the nervous system is the spinal nerves. These are the nerves connected to the spinal cord. The cervical, brachial, thoracic, lumbar and sacral spinal nerves form separate nerve plexuses (groups of nerves). Each nerve plexus distributes electricity into certain areas of the body, through the peripheral nerves, which are the nerves that travel from the spinal nerves throughout the entire body. When testing each nerve plexus, the spinal nerves connected to that plexus are what are being tested. If that particular plexus is not working at least sufficiently, then there is a problem in one or more of the spinal nerves connected to that particular plexus.

"Are all nerve plexuses working perfectly?"

If not, test which plexus is not working perfectly. There could be more than one. The spinal nerve plexuses are cervical plexus, brachial plexus, thoracic plexus, lumbar plexus and sacral plexus. Since the above question tested false, one or more of the plexuses won't be functioning perfectly. A nerve plexus can test underactive or overactive. If the plexus is not working perfectly, it has to be one or the other. All you have to do is ask;

"Is this nerve plexus functioning at least sufficiently?"

If the answer is "yes", the plexus is overactive. If it tests "no", the problem is causing the plexus to be underactive.

"Is the cervical plexus working perfectly? brachial plexus? thoracic plexus? lumbar plexus? sacral plexus?"

If the answer is "yes," for the first cervical plexus, continue naming each plexus until you test a weakness. Next, test the spinal nerves connected to that particular plexus, and correct the imbalance. When that spinal nerve is corrected, re-test that plexus to confirm energy is flowing perfectly. Once the first spinal nerve is corrected, and the plexus is still not functioning perfectly, there is another spinal nerve, in that plexus, that needs to be corrected. When that plexus tests strong, repeat the first question to make sure all plexuses are working perfectly.

The reason nerve plexuses are important is they distribute all of the electrical energy/information from the brain to the body, and body to the brain. The spinal cord is the conduit for this energy, and each spinal nerve that is connected is distributing energy to its assigned parts of the body.

Autonomic Nervous System

All of the involuntary body functions such as breathing, heartbeat, hormone production, immune system response, and blood pressure are controlled by the autonomic nervous system. A good way to remember it is think "automatic" nervous system. It is divided in to two different groups of nerves – parasympathetic and sympathetic.

The sympathetic nerves can be compared to the accelerator in the car. It controls of some areas of the body and slows down some other areas. Over active sympathetic nerves result in the fight-flight or flee. The condition is referred to as "sympathetic dominant,or mode" It is triggered by the limbic system in the brain reacting to some type of stimuli and interpreting it as fear.

"Is the autonomic nervous system balanced?"

If "no," ask;

"Are the sympathetic nerves out of balance?"

"Are the parasympathetic nerves balanced?"

Wherever the cause is found, test if the reason is a toxin, parasite, nutritional deficiency and/ or tissue damage. Correct it with a supplement in the Appendix.

Peripheral Nerves

The peripheral nerves carry the energy from the nerve plexuses, to all the organs, and glands of the body. The nerves that carry commands from the brain to the body are the motor or efferent nerves. These nerves are responsible for every action of the body. Without motor nerves giving the orders to the muscles, they couldn't move. This transmission of energy is innervation.

There is also information constantly being sent to the brain through the afferent, or sensory nerves. The body doesn't know what a stimulus means until the brain deciphers the message, and sends it back as a response. Cutaneous nerves are located closest to the skin. They are responsible for tactile stimuli.

"Motor nerves are free of inflammation and not causing any of this symptom."

"Innervation is flowing perfectly."

"Sensory nerves are free of inflammation and functioning perfectly."

"Cutaneous nerves are free of inflammation and not causing this symptom."

Nerve function needs to be muscle tested for "perfect". The reason is, if you test "at least sufficient," if the nerve is over active, the muscle tests strong, not telling you there are overactive tissue causing the problem. But, if you ask if the nerve tissue is working "perfectly" and it is not, then you ask;

"Is this nerve functioning under 100%?"

With this one simple question, you know whether the tissue is underactive, or over active. This technique can be used with any tissue, not just nerves. Whichever it is, find the functioning percentage and root cause. Refer to the Appendix to select the correct supplement.

If you are experiencing numbness, or sharp pain, it is very possibly the sensory nerves. The cause of numbness is the sensory nerves are underactive, and not able to deliver the stimuli to the brain. If the symptom is sharp pain, the sensory nerves are being over stimulated, usually because of a heavy metal or ionic heavy metal toxin.

If movement is the problem, the motor nerves are usually the culprit. If there is a difficulty of weakness, or loss of control, it is the motor nerves. Twitching is a symptom of overactivated motor nerves.

Inflamed cutaneous nerves cause itching, and pain. These "surface" nerves are involved in skin rashes, irritation, and inflammation. Shingle breakouts are in the cutaneous nerves.

Anxiety is often caused by a lack of calcium in the nerves. This happens especially to women. If you are suffering from nervousness, or anxiety, consider calcium, and B complex vitamins. You can find out if you need it by asking;

"Is the calcium in the nerves sufficient?"

"Are all B vitamins sufficient?"

"Are either a calcium or B vitamin deficiency causing this anxiety, or nervousness?"

The first two questions should test strong, and the third question should test weak, if you are healthy in these areas. If the third question tests "yes", ask;

"Is a calcium deficiency causing this symptom?"

If the answer is "yes", you have determined there is a calcium deficiency, but don't stop there. There could also be a B complex deficiency also. Ask;

"Is there also a B Complex deficiency?"

In muscle testing it is important to be aware of how you ask the question. Sometimes the correct answer is a strong arm. If a question is asked differently, then the correct answer will be a weak response. The above three questions illustrate this concept.

Sensory Organs

The last part of the nervous system is the sensory organs – eyes and ears.

The Eyes

The eyes are an extension of the brain. These sensory organs are complex. The best way to test the eyes is by asking;

"Are the eyes working at least sufficiently?" or "Are the eyes causing any of this particular problem?"

Dry eyes are a common ailment, that is associated with the lacrimal apparatus. Ask;

"Is the lacrimal apparatus causing dry eyes?"

If the answer is "yes", continue testing to find the part of the lacrimal apparatus causing the problem.

"Are the lacrimal glands causing the dryness?, the lacrimal sacs, and/or lacrimal ducts?"

Each of these areas can be tested if there is a concern with dry eyes. There can be more than one reason. Keep testing the original question, until there are no more reasons for dryness in the eyes.

If the arm stays strong test the different parts of the lacrimal apparatus. If "no," test;

"Is the root cause of dry eyes in the eyes?"

If "yes", further testing of the different parts of the eye should be done. If the answer is "no", locate the system that is causing the problem, and correct it. After balancing the first cause, always test the original question to see if there are any other reasons.

Poor vision is assumed to be a natural progression of aging. The only answer is a prescription for glasses. It is true, they will help a person see better, but like all prescriptions, glasses don't address the root cause of why the person's eyesight is not 20/20.

Normal visual perception is controlled by the ocular motor system.

"Is the ocular motor system working sufficiently in both eyes?"

If the muscle response is weak, and a decline of vision is a concern, test the ciliary muscles. These muscles control "accommodation", which is the adjustment of the lens.

"Is accommodation of near and far sightedness functioning at least sufficiently?"

"Are the ciliary muscles functioning at least sufficiently?"

"Is the lens causing the vision problem?"

The lens is designed to change shape as we view objects at different distances. The lens nutrition is supplied by the aqueous humor. It is crucial for the lens to have sufficient water, and nutrients. To find out ask;

"Is water sufficient in the lens?"

"Are there any nutritional deficiencies in the lens?"

Cataracts are a build-up of protein on the lens, which causes a distortion in the lens. Most people who develop cataracts have surgery. The lens is removed and a new lens is replaced. If you discover a cataract forming on your lens, by correcting the problem early can be corrected.

"Are both lens free of cataracts?"

Glaucoma is the result of excess pressure inside the eyeball. Fluids are constantly flowing in, and out of this hollow sphere. A delicate balance of flow is crucial to keep the correct pressure in the eye to sustain its shape. When the eye is not draining at the same rate as fluid enters, the pressure of the eye increases. This is diagnosed as glaucoma. Insevere cases the excess pressure damages the optic nerve which can cause blindness. In most cases it is an adhesion, not allowing the fluid to drain properly.

"Is both eyes ocular pressure normal? In range?

If the answer is "no", ask;

"Is it because of an adhesion?"

If "yes", refer to the Appendix for the recommended supplement. If "no" ask;

"Is the root cause of this high ocular pressure in the eye?"

If "yes", continue testing the other parts of the eye. If "no", muscle test for what system the root cause is located, and continue the protocol.

Here are two stories about my wife, Ann. A few years ago, Ann went to the eye doctor and she was alarmed because Ann had high eye pressure. The doctor diagnosed it as glaucoma, and tried to prescribe a medication. Ann refused, informing the doctor, "My husband is a Naturopath doctor. He will take care of it." Ann returned to the same office for her next yearly checkup, and the doctor didn't even mention glaucoma!

Ann damaged her eye with a contact, causing severe eye pain. She was referred to an eye specialist, who after an exam, started writing out two different prescriptions. I asked him, "would you tell me what is the actual problem?" He explained to me Ann had ripped cells off her sclera, the white part of the eye. I started wondering why those cells would have ripped. There had to be a reason and there was.

We left the eye doctors office with our two prescriptions, that we never filled. I muscle tested the reason was a deficiency of Vitamin C, and citrus bioflavonoids. I started Ann on a high dose for the two weeks before returning to the doctor. He was pleased with her progress, and told us, "Just keep doing what you're doing." We followed the doctor's orders, and kept doing the Vitamin C, and citrus bioflavonoids, for another two weeks. The eye was healed perfectly, and there was never a prescription drug taken. The doctor never knew it.

There is no natural eye exam available through the normal eye care facilities. This program offers a proven system, that can help you achieve better eyesight. The eyes are the "windows" of the soul." Take care of them.

The Ears

Vertigo, tinnitus, and loss of hearing, are the main complaints concerning the auditory.

The three main areas of the ear are the outer canal, mid-ear, and inner ear. The eardrum separates the outer ear, and the mid-ear. The ossicles – malleus, incus, and stapes, are located in the mid-ear. The inner ear contains the cochlea, and the semi-circular canals. These semi-circular canals are where the root cause of vertigo will be found. To test for problems in the ear start by asking;

"Is the root cause in the outer ear? mid-ear? inner ear?

Find the section of the ear where the root cause is located. If it is in the mid-ear ask;

"Is the root problem in the malleus (hammer)? incus (anvil)? stapes (stirrup)? Oval window

If the root cause is in the inner ear ask;

"Is the root cause in the semi-circular canals? cochlea? Vestibulocochlear nerve?"

The vestibulocochlear nerve is the cranial nerve that transmits auditory stimuli to the brain.

If any of these questions answer weak, refer to the assessment sheet, and test for what system the problem is located. Muscle test the ears and eyes just like any other organ or gland. The sensory organs, like all the organs and glands are complex. If the reader desires more information refer to an anatomy book.

This concludes the nervous system. Remember, the brain communicates with every cell, tissue, organ and gland. Without the nervous system, there would be no connection. Without the brain, there would be no "command center." Without the peripheral nerves the body could not send stimuli to the brain, or relay information back to the systems of the body. Whenever there is a health symptom always test the nervous system.

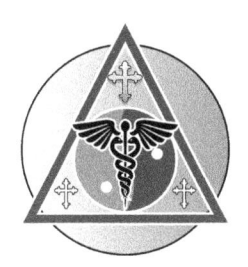

CHAPTER TWELVE

The Respiratory System – Your Oxygen Deliverer

How long can you live without oxygen? All of us know how important the respiratory system is. Yet, we take it for granted as it tirelessly works every day, delivering fresh oxygen to our bodies and eliminating harmful carbon dioxide. We take approximately 20,000 breaths every day and don't think about it – until something goes wrong.

Sinus congestion, headache, cough, fatigue, asthma type conditions, and shortness of breath are symptoms of a problem in the respiratory system.

The respiratory system is divided into the upper respiratory - the paranasal sinus, and the lower respiratory, which includes the bronchi and lungs.

Upper Respiratory (Paranasal Sinus)

Sinus congestion is a common ailment. Sinuses are cavities, lined with mucosa. When this tissue becomes irritated by toxins or parasites, it gets inflamed and swells. This swelling makes breathing through the nostrils difficult. The pressure, from this swelling, can cause headaches. To decide what part of the respiratory system is causing a symptom, ask;

"Is the "root cause" of this symptom in the upper respiratory tract."

If the answer is "no," start testing the lower respiratory system. If the answer is "yes," you are getting closer to the root cause. You don't have to test the lower respiratory system. The body has already told you that the first cause of the symptom is in the upper respiratory. The next step is to locate the root cause in the paranasal sinuses. Ask;

"Is the root cause in the mucosal lining of the paranasal cavity?"

The paranasal sinuses are cavities inside the skull. If the problem is in the sinuses, in most cases it will be in the mucosal lining of the sinuses. The sections of the paranasal sinus are maxillary sinus, which are located in the upper cheek areas, the ethmoid sinus, which is located between and around the eyes. The frontal sinus is located above the eyes in the forehead area. If you want to be more accurate, once you determine the root cause is in the paranasal sinus, ask;

"Is the root cause in the mucosal lining of the maxillary? ethmoid? frontal?"

There are other sinuses in the head. Dural venous sinuses travel across the top of the head. There are also sinuses in the back of the head. Inflammation and swelling of the mucosal lining from any of these sinuses can cause headaches, pressure, and pain.

"Is the root cause in the Dural venous sinuses?"

"Is the issue in the sinuses in the occipital lobe area?"

If this question tests true, the next step is to first test for functioning then the root cause. Rebalance the area using the Appendix.

Lower Respiratory System

Air travels down the trachea (windpipe) into the bronchioles and throughout the lungs. Carbon dioxide is exhaled through the lungs and oxygen is supplied by the lungs. Once you have established the root cause of the health problem is in the lower respiratory muscle test each option in the lower respiratory system.

"Is the root cause in the trachea?"

"Is the root cause in the bronchi?

"Is the root cause in the lungs?"

"Is the root cause in the diaphragm?"

Receiving a true strong muscle response signals that the root cause is in that portion of the respiratory system. After correcting the first root cause retest all the options to be certain there isn't a second reason. If you test that there is a second reason retest again to determine if there is a third reason. Continue this fashion until there are no other reason in the respiratory system. Don't ever assume there is only one reason for the stress inducing the symptom. The only way to know for sure is to muscle test.

Coughs are usually in the bronchioles but can be caused by something in the lungs. To be more precise there are the primary, secondary, tertiary and higher order bronchioles. As a general muscle "bronchioles" will produce a general answer. To be more specific each section of bronchioles should be tested.

"Is the root cause in the primary? secondary? tertiary? higher order bronchioles?"

The right and left lung should be tested for cough or lack of breath. The bronchioles are inside the lungs but both of them muscle test separately. To get a complete answer for cough or lack of breath both areas of the respiratory system should be tested.

"Is the right or left lung causing this issue?"

Some reasons for coughs are virus, mildew, mold, environmental toxins and/or carcinogens. All of these possible causes by asking the body;

"Is the reason in the lungs a virus? ildew? mold, environmental toxins, etc?"

Once the root cause is found refer to the SSR section to find the correct supplement.

Asthma type of symptoms can be caused by many factors. Dehydration is a leading cause. When a person cannot get their breath the alveoli (air sacs) should be tested. These grape looking bunches are responsible for the oxygen-gas exchange. When the alveoli are not working properly, they are either "closed shut" or "stuck open". If they are closed the root cause is always in the bronchioles, which attach to the alveoli.

"Are the alveoli functioning perfectly?"

If "no;" ask;

"Are the alveoli causing this breathing issue?"

If "yes;"

Are the alveoli closed?"

If they are closed it is because of parasitic activity in the bronchioles. If they are stuck open it is an adhesion. Refer to the SSR how to remove the adhesion. Refer to the parasitic chart to find the type of parasite and how to kill it.

The Diaphragm

Another part of the lower respiratory system is the diaphragm. These are the muscles that are critical for inhalation and exhalation. If either inhalation or exhalation is not functioning sufficiently check the diaphragm. If the reason is in these muscles but the root cause is not in the diaphragm then test the phrenic nerve. This part of the vagus nerve controls the innervation to the diaphragm.

"Is the diaphragm is causing this problem?"

"Is the root cause in the diaphragm?"

If the problem is the diaphragm but the root cause is not in the muscle test for innervation – electrical flow.

"Innervation to the diaphragm is perfect?"

If it is not flowing perfectly test the phrenic nerve.

"Is the root cause in the phrenic nerve?"

This concludes the chapter on the respiratory system. We have covered the upper and lower respiratory system. Breath is life. We come in to this world with our first breath, and we depart with our last breath. The respiratory system provides every breath we take. Be grateful, and don't take this life saving system for granted.

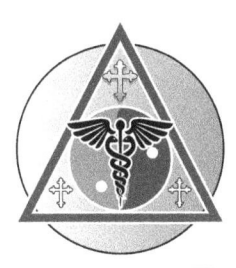

CHAPTER THIRTEEN

The Reproductive System – The Giver of Life

As human beings we are designed to reproduce. Our purpose is to create life. The reproductive system gives us the means for a miracle – to create human life. It is also the system that supplies the steroid hormones, such as progesterone, estrogens, and testosterone.

More problems are happening in the reproductive system as our environment gets poisoned with toxins. Women are having difficulty with monthly periods, infertility, hot flashes, mood swings and night sweats. Because of xenoestrogens (fake estrogen from foods and environment), male sperm has drastically plummeted.

As we age our hormones decline, causing other issues such as premature aging, fatigue, lack of cognitive skills, loss of bone density, and low libido. The reproductive system and hormones are still important, even if you are over childbearing years. It is important for bone strength and is critical for muscle firmness, mood and sex drive. The better your reproductive system is functioning, the younger and more vital your body will feel.

Female Reproductive System

The ovaries are the gonads, or sexual glands of a female. The ovaries are responsible for the production of progesterone, estrogens, and testosterone. There are three different estrogen hormones – estrone (E1), estradiol (E2), and estriol (E3). Estradiol and estriol are beneficial for the body and anti-cancerous. Estrone is not beneficial for the body and can be harmful.

These hormones are controlled through the HPA axis – the hypothalamus, pituitary, adrenal axis. This is the cascade which feeds the ovaries the required hormones. The process starts in the hypothalamus, where the follicle stimulating releasing hormone and the luteinizing releasing hormones are made, and secreted to the anterior pituitary gland. The anterior pituitary gland produces, and secretes the follicle stimulating hormone (FSH), and the luteinizing hormone (LH) to the gonads. The ovaries can't make the steroid hormones sufficiently, if they don't receive the correct hormones from the anterior pituitary. To make sure these areas are functioning sufficiently ask;

"Is the hypothalamus producing all "releasing hormones" to the anterior pituitary sufficiently?"

"Is the anterior pituitary releasing all hormones sufficiently to the ovaries?"

"Are the ovaries *receiving* all hormones from the pituitary?"

If any of these questions answer weak (no), look for the root cause, and rebalance the offending tissue.

If you are experiencing pain in the frontal lower abdomen, it could be the ovaries.

"Are the ovaries causing this pain?"

"Are the ovaries *producing* hormones sufficiently?"

"Are the ovaries free of inflammation?"

The right and left ovary are connected to the uterus by the right and left fallopian tubes. When an egg is released in the ovary, thousands of sperm travel up the fallopian tubes to intercept the egg, which starts the fertilization process. One egg is released each month of the menstrual cycle during ovulation. The release of the egg alternates between the two ovaries.

"Are both ovaries releasing an egg perfectly?"

"Are the fallopian tubes working perfectly?"

Once the egg has been fertilized, it attaches to the uterine wall. The most important hormone at this time of the early pregnancy is progesterone. If progesterone is low, the fetus cannot be carried, and will result in a miscarriage.

"Is progesterone perfect in the uterine lining?"

"Is the uterus perfect in hormones?"

If you are experiencing cramping this is usually the smooth muscle of the cervix or uterine wall. Often, magnesium is low because of either lack of intake, or not being utilized properly.

"Is the reason for this cramping found in the smooth muscle of the cervix? Uterus?

Is it being caused by a magnesium deficiency?"

"Can magnesium be utilized in this tissue at this time?"

If the test states "yes", add magnesium to your diet. If it can't be utilized, then check magnesium receptors in that tissue.

"Are the magnesium receptors working sufficiently?

If "no," test to find the root cause why the magnesium receptors are stopping the magnesium from being used. Many times, a lack of magnesium of the smooth muscles of the uterus or fibromuscular tissue of the cervix is deficient in magnesium. Refer to the Appendix to find the correct supplement to remove the toxin, and then test to make sure magnesium can be utilized. Once magnesium can be utilized perfectly, test that the amount of magnesium will now be optimum, or at least sufficient, after taking the chosen supplement.

Caution: Taking too much magnesium will cause the stools of the bowel to become too soft. This is a sign of bowel intolerance of magnesium. Reduce, or stop magnesium until the bowels are back to normal.

Vaginal tissue is susceptible to yeast infections. Candida Albicans (yeast) love this area. To counter this attack, make sure that the microbiome, in the vaginal canal, is sufficient. Probiotics are as important for the vaginal tissue as they are for the gut.

Vaginal pain can be caused by atrophy, which is the wasting away of the tissue. This is caused by a deficiency of estrogen. Another reason for vaginal pain is lack of secretion. To find out if either of these issues is involved, ask;

"Is the root cause of this vaginal pain (or itching) in the vagina tissue?"

"Is this vaginal pain being caused by atrophy?

If "yes;"

"Is it because of a lack of estrogen?"

If "no;"

"Is it because of a lack of secretion?"

Proceed and test for a toxin, parasite, nutritional deficiency, or tissue damage. If there is tissue damage, there is a reason why the tissue was damaged. Always remember, there can be multiple reasons for the same symptom. Just because an estrogen deficiency tested that it caused the atrophy, does not mean there isn't possibly a mineral or vitamin deficiency. Always test "is there another reason for this issue?"

If yes, refer to Appendix for supplement recommendation. Once you select the correct supplement, muscle test if the chosen supplement is beneficial toward the problem

Concerns about their breasts, such as fibroid cysts, sore breasts, lumps and cancer are being experienced by millions of women. Many of these symptoms are caused by a lack of iodine, a misfunctioning lymph system, and/or estrogen dominance.

Most Americans do not receive adequate iodine. In the states, where there is no oceans, the iodine supply is low. Iodine is the most important nutrient the thyroid needs to make thyroid hormones. The health department's answer was to fortify table salt with iodine. But, the catch 22 is that to receive the amount of iodine needed, high doses of table salt would need to be taken. The issue with that idea is that table salt is not healthy for our bodies. It causes damage to the artery lining, and creates high blood pressure.

Lymph flow is crucial for healthy breasts. There are many lymph nodes under each armpit, which influence the health of the breasts. The "micro lymph" brings the waste from the cells and tissue. It includes the lymph capillaries, afferent lymph vessels, lymph nodes, and afferent lymph vessels. The micro lymph drains into the macro lymph system. The most important areas to test in the macro lymph are the left and right lymph duct, the thoracic lymph duct and the cisterna chyli.

One reason for breast soreness is excess estrogen. This is estrogen dominance. The reason is an imbalance of the progesterone to estrogen ratio. This ratio can be measured through muscle testing. The minimum the ratio should be is 10 progesterone to 1 estrogen. Maximum and optimal health is 20 progesterone to 1 estrogen.

In today's environment there are many "fake" estrogens in our meats, dairy, water and plastics. We are immersed in a sea of estrogen. These "estrogens" - called xenoestrogens, enter the body acting like real estrogen. This imbalance causes hot flashes, sore breasts, large hips, and even breast cancer.

"Are the breasts free of growths? fibroid cysts? calcium deposits? fat deposits?"

If the answer is "no",

"Is it because of an iodine deficiency? Is iodine beneficial?"

"Is it being caused by the lymph system?"

"Is the cause estrogen dominance?"

If you do notice a growth in your breast, contact your health care practitioner. As a Naturopath doctor, I don't suggest mammograms. They are not as accurate as people believe, they place too much pressure on the breasts, and add more toxic radiation into your body. I do suggest thermography. A credible muscle tester can find the problem and be less invasive. You can find the problem yourself using this system of muscle testing that you are holding in your hands. That is how close the answers are.

These questions that you are learning can be asked about any tissue. More than one answer is possible. **Always look for the number one primary reason. After you have corrected that imbalance, test all of the areas again to make sure there is not another problem in the system.**

Male Reproductive System

Men don't want to admit it, but are suffering from many reproductive system issues such as ED, swollen prostates, high PSA, low testosterone and lack of sex drive. Because of excess xenoestrogens (fake estrogen), which mimic estrogen in the body, men have experienced a feminizing of the body, which includes lower testosterone and less potent sperm.

Both men and women have estrogen, but estrogen is higher in women than men. When males start building up too much estrogen, the body starts changing. This is due to the accumulation of xenoestrogens in meats, water and plastics. To find out if you have too much estrogen ask;

"Is the blood free of xenoestrogens?"

If "no," why?

"Is the liver detoxing xenoestrogens perfectly?"

"Can the nephrons of the kidneys filter out all xenoestrogen?"

If "no," why? Repair the problem in the kidneys, before you clean the blood of xenoestrogens. Once the kidneys are filtering perfectly, it's time to detox the excess estrogen. Refer to the Appendix for the correct supplement.

Another reason men's hormones are declining is too much testosterone is aromatizing. When this happens, testosterone is converted to a harmful estrogen, which accumulates, and eventually causes disease, including cancer. It also decreases natural testosterone, which decreases sex drive, ambition and contributes to muscle loss. Aromatization is caused by a deficiency of zinc. It is estimated 75% of Americans are deficient in zinc.

"Is testosterone aromatizing into harmful estrogen?"

If "yes," ask;

"Is it because of zinc deficiency?"

If this test is true, find out why there is a zinc deficiency. Is it because of the deficiency of zinc in the diet? Can it be utilized properly by the cells?" Does a zinc supplement make the above statement go false, which means that supplement or food will correct the zinc deficiency?

The main focus for men should be the prostate. A majority of men over fifty have swollen prostates. The cause for this swelling is toxins such as cadmium, nickel, and other heavy metal toxins. Zinc and selenium are important nutrients for the health of the prostate. Saw Palmetto is a well - known herb for prostate health, and is always beneficial.

If a man is having frequent urination, and dribbling there is a good chance there are problems in the prostate.

Questions that can be used to test the male reproductive system are;

"Is the prostate free of inflammation?"

"Is the prostate free of swelling?

"Is the prostate free of heavy metal toxins?"

"Is the penis receiving sufficient blood flow?"

"Are the testicles producing testosterone sufficiently?"

E.D. are dreadful letters for any man. Just the thought of not being able to perform "like a man" can be devastating. Just like any true root cause, the reason is not always the same. Every case must be muscle tested through the system to find the root causes. The following are some of the questions that will help pinpoint the problem.

"Is this problem caused by a physical imbalance?

If "yes," start by asking the following question. If "no," ask if it is emotional.

"Is the ED caused by a lack of blood flow?"

If the primary reason is blood flow, refer to the Circulatory section.

If no, muscle test for the tissue causing the ED such as;

"Is the tissue causing this symptom functioning at 90% or better? If the answer is "no" ask; "80% or better.

Continue counting down until you get a strong arm, then increase by twos until the arm goes weak. Once that tissue is found, muscle test for which of the four reason is causing the condition – toxins, nutritional deficiency, parasite, or tissue damage. After you correct the first imbalance, test again to find any other issues causing the condition. Continue testing until there are no other reasons at this time.

Remember; Muscle testing is a tool to communicate with the body. The body's intelligence will tell you what needs to be done at this time. Don't be surprised when after you fix what you thought was everything, and then you discover something else. There are layers of healing. You can only test what the body tells you. Your job is to perform an accurate, nonbiased, muscle test, and allow the body to communicate to you what it needs.

In this, or any health crisis there can trapped or repressed emotional components involved. Refer to either <u>The Emotion Code</u> by Dr. Bradley Nelson or Emotional Release Therapy, which is part of the Body Balance Healing System and discussed later in the book.

This concludes the reproductive system.

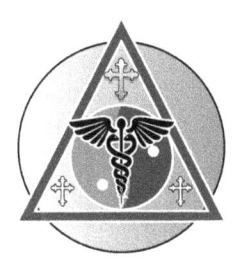

CHAPTER FOURTEEN

The Structural System – The Foundation

Without the structural system the body would have no shape. It would be a blob of tissue that couldn't move. Without bones, joints, muscles, connective tissue, cartilage fasciae and skin the body wouldn't have a frame. These are the components of the structural system.

Bones

The bones are the strength of the framework. They shape the body and protect the inner organs from damage. The bones produce the red blood cells (erythrocytes) and white blood cells (leucocytes) in the bone marrow.

The major disease of the bones is osteoporosis which translates to "holes in the bone". To a lesser degree is the beginning of osteoporosis – osteopenia. Both of these terms relate to loss of bone density. Osteopenia is the start of this loss and osteoporosis is more severe.

These issues can be stopped and possibly reversed with the correct nutrients. This is *not* just a deficiency of calcium. This is what medical doctors have been prescribing for years. If that was the "cure" there should be no osteoporosis. The truth is there is more osteoporosis and osteopenia today. Why? Because the root cause is not being addressed.

What is the root cause? The only way to dig deeper and find the answer is with muscle testing.

"Is the bone density (check wrist, hip bones and/or spine) perfect?"

The density of the bone needs to be perfect, not sufficient. Any bone density less than 98% is osteoporosis by medical testing standards. One of the primary reasons for lack of density is the imbalance of osteoblast and osteoclast cells.

The osteoblast and osteoclast cells remodel the bone. Osteoclast cells dissolve old worn out bone and osteoblast cells rebuild new bone. An imbalance in either one eventually creates disease in the bones.

"Are the osteoclasts and osteoblasts balanced?"

If they are not balanced just ask why;

"Why are they not balanced?" "toxin?" "parasite?" "nutritional deficiency?" "tissue damage?"

The answer should be one or more of these. Once you select what is causing the problem refer to the SSR to correct it. Hormone imbalance of progesterone and estrogen can also cause loss of bone density. Ask;

"Is estrogen or progesterone causing any of this bone loss?"

If the answer is yes then ask;

"Is a deficiency of estrogen causing this problem?"

"Is a deficiency of progesterone causing this issue?"

If either or both are deficient refer to the Appendix in the hormone section.

Joints

Joints are structures that connect bone to bone. Without joints the body could not move in the various manners. There are many types of joints in the body. In this book the word "joint" will refer to all joints. If more precise testing of a particular joint is desired please refer to an anatomy atlas.

"Is a joint causing this symptom?"

If "yes," test the synovial fluid. This is the lubrication of the joints. It is secreted from the synovial membrane.

"Is it caused by a deficiency in synovial fluid?"

If "no," follow normal testing procedures. If "yes," then the root cause is in the synovial membrane. Fix the synovial membrane, the synovial fluid will be perfect. After correcting this imbalance ask;

"Is there another reason in the joints that are causing this symptom?"

Many conventional medical doctors diagnose a patient with "arthritis." This is not a helpful diagnosis. The word "arthritis" means "inflammation of the joints." This medical diagnosis tells the patient nothing that s/he didn't know already. The real answer is to find the root cause of *why there is inflammation in the joint.*

Some of the reason for inflammation in the joints are dehydration, burrulia bergdorferi (Lyme disease), deficiency of essential fatty acids, acidic ph, nutritional deficiency, and/or toxins. If there is inflammation of the joints tests these possible reasons. Also test for the four main reasons for stress in the joints and refer to the Appendix.

Muscles

Without muscles the body could not move. Every movement, from a blink of an eye, a heartbeat or breath takes an elaborate system of muscles to do what we take for granted. Muscles give our body tone and strength. To find out if the muscles are causing any of the health concern ask;

"Is this health issue caused by muscles?"

If "yes," find which muscles by ask;

"Is the root cause of this problem in the skeletal muscles? smooth muscles? cardiac muscles?"

Once the particular group of muscles are found proceed through testing the functioning, and reason. For the more advanced use the Fingerprinting program to find the root cause. If you are not using the Fingerprinting procedures which are taught in Chapter Seventeen use the basic four reasons. Refer to SSR.

There are three types of muscles. Skeletal muscles are the muscles that are used to move the body such as walking, standing, or exercising. These are voluntary muscles which means that we control their movement. The second type is smooth muscles. These muscles are involuntary being controlled by the autonomic nervous system. We do not have any control on these muscles. They are located inside the blood vessels, lungs, GI tract and more. All of them are working and we don't even know it. The third type of muscle is the cardiac muscles. These muscles are found exclusively in the heart.

Connective Tissue

Connected to the joints are ligaments which support the joints. They are bands of fibrous connective tissue that connect bones to bones and keeps the joints in place. Ligaments also support and maintain organs. Tendons and ligaments are similar because they are both connective tissue but tendons connect bones to muscles. The third type of connective tissue is fasciae which connects muscles to muscles.

If any of these connective tissues are causing the issue test for the basic reasons of toxins, parasites, nutritional deficiency or tissue damage. To locate which connective tissue is causing the problem ask;

"Is this symptom being caused by a ligament? tendon? fasciae?"

As in all tissue, find where the root cause is located, determine the cause and refer to SSR to correct the imbalance. Always check if there is a secondary problem to the symptom.

Fascia

Fascia is connective tissue between the skin and the muscle. It surrounds every organ, gland and tissue throughout the complete body, from head to toe. The three layers of fascia are the superficial, deep and visceral fascia. To find out if the fascia is the root cause of the health concern, ask;

"Is the fascia causing this symptom?"

If the answer is yes, ask;

"Is it the superficial? deep? visceral?"

It could be more than one layer of fascia causing the problem. Once the first area of the fascia is corrected, again repeat the questions again about the fascia and continue until the fascia tests strong.

Skin

The skin is the largest organ of the body. It serves to protect us from harmful environmental antagonists. It is the outer covering of our body. It helps regulate body temperature. It holds everything together. The skin is part of the elimination process. The skin is an important component of the health puzzle.

The skin has many layers stacked on top of each other. The top group of layers is the epidermis. It is composed of the basement membrane, stratum basale, stratum spinosum, stratum granulosum, stratum lucidum and stratum corneum. When the root cause is in the skin ask;

"Is the primary cause in the epithelium (upper group)?

If "yes," test each stratum (layer);

"Is the root cause in the stratum basale? stratum spinosum? Stratum granulosum? Stratum lucidum; or stratum corneum?"

Soft tissue is the tissue under the skin that forms the cushion for the body. Soft tissue doesn't muscle test the same as skin so it does need to be tested separately.

"The root cause is in the soft tissue?"

If there is a problem in this area find the root cause and correct it using the Appendix.

Remember that there can be more than one area causing the symptom, Start with the primary root cause. Correct the primary cause and then muscle test to see if there is a secondary or tertiary cause. Always continue testing for another cause for the symptom until the body tells you there are no more causes for that particular symptom at this time.

If the body tests no, proceed to the dermis which is where the action of the skin takes place. If it has been established through muscle testing that the root cause is in the skin and it is *not* in the upper layers it has to be in the dermis. The dermis contains the blood vessels, nerve endings, melanocyte cells, which supply skin pigment, hair follicles, sweat glands and oil glands.

"Is the root cause in the dermis?"

When it originally tests that the root cause is in the skin but not in the upper layers the answer has to be in the dermis. Once that the root cause is determined to be in the dermis muscle test each component of the dermis. Refer to an anatomy book to see a section of the dermis and test every part of the dermis to locate the root cause of the health issue.

The structural system is an important part of the natural health assessment. Acne, rash, and itching are some of the symptoms of a skin issue. In Chinese medicine the skin is referred to as the "third kidney." When there are physical stress showing in the skin the blood has toxins, which is caused by either the liver not detoxing perfectly or the nephrons in the kidneys not filtering all the toxins or both. When either one of these don't function perfectly the skin is the part of the body that gets stressed and shows the symptom.

Most skin issues are *not* skin issues. The root cause is deeper. I feel sorry for dermatologists, who try to heal the problem with topical creams, and laser, but never examine the deeper core reason. You can muscle test and find out if the problem is truly in the skin;

"Is the root cause in the skin?"

If "no," ask;

"Is the root cause of this skin issue in the liver? nephrons? kidneys?"

These are the three main areas that will cause skin problems. If none of these three are the root cause, muscle test which system the root cause is located.

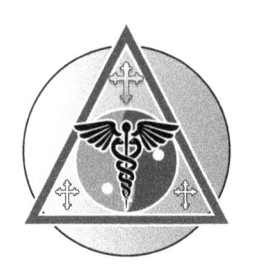

CHAPTER FIFTEEN

The Urinary System – Your Balancer

The main part of the excretory system is the urinary system. It consists of an upper, and lower section. The upper urinary system is the kidneys and ureters. The lower urinary system consists of the bladder and urethra. The urinary system keeps the body fluids balanced, by secreting excess nutrients and toxins from the body and reabsorbing what is needed by the body.

The most common complaints in the urinary system are UTI (urinary tract infection), incontinence, edema, and frequency of urination. All of these can be corrected naturally.

Upper Urinary System

Once the urinary system muscle tests as the system containing the root cause, start by asking;

"Is the root cause (whatever the complaint is) in the upper urinary system?"

If it is true, the root cause is in either the kidneys, ureters, or both. If it is false, then the root cause is in either the bladder, urethra, or both. If it is in the upper part start by asking;

"Is the root cause in the kidneys?"

The first thing to check is blood flow into both kidneys. Ask;

"Is blood flow sufficient in both kidneys?"

If blood flow is not sufficient, test the renal arteries. Ask;

"Is blood flow into both kidneys through the renal arteries functioning at least sufficiently?"

"If not, refer to the circulatory chapter and test what area of the artery is causing the problem.

The kidneys are the main filtration station. A million nephrons are contained in each kidney, filter toxins, and reabsorb nutrients, and water. If the cause is in the kidneys ask;

"Is the root cause in the nephrons?"

To get more specific in muscle testing, refer to an anatomy book and test each individual area in the nephrons. This is a more precise test than just testing "nephrons."

If the kidneys are the source of the root cause, but is not in the nephrons test;

"Is the root cause in the cortex of the kidneys?"

If the root cause is in the upper urinary, and not in the kidneys, then it is in the ureters. Confirm by asking;

"Is the primary cause in the ureters?"

If the problem is in the ureters, test for stones, tissue damage or adhesions.

"Are the ureters free of stones? tissue damage? adhesions?"

Lower Urinary System

If the answer is the lower half of the urinary system, ask;

"Is the root cause in the bladder?"

If the answer is "yes," find the root cause in that tissue, and correct the imbalance.

To check the bladder, muscle test the functioning of the smooth muscle, trigone, If the answer is no then ask;

"Is the root cause in the urethra?"

One reason for excess frequency of urination is the bladder not emptying totally. The bladder is like a pouch that fills up with urine. When the bladder fills, the detrusor muscle fibers are signaled to contract, which pushes the urine out of the bladder and into the urethra. But if the detrusor muscle fibers are not working perfectly there will be urine left in the bladder.

"Is the bladder emptying perfectly?"

If "no," ask;

"Is the reason in the detrusor muscle fibers?"

"Is the cause in the urethra."

After correcting the "primary" root cause, always test if there is a "secondary" reason for the problem in that same system. If the answer is no, then ask;

"Are there any other reasons for this symptom in any oth system?"

If "yes," start at the top of the assessment sheet, and work down until the system that has the next cause is found. If "no," focus on the next symptom by starting a new test.

Urinary tract infections (UTI) are a common urinary problem. This happens when infection is present in the bladder. This can also create frequent bathroom visits. The most common culprit for this is pathological bacteria, which are non-beneficial bacteria which creates infection. To decide if this is the problem, ask;

"Is the bladder free of infection?"

If "no," ask;

"Is the cause pathological bacteria?"

If "no," refer to the parasite charts in the Appendix, and select the parasite that is causing the infection.

If "yes," refer to the parasite chart and find pathological bacteria (bacteria) and test the suggested supplement. If that supplement doesn't test strong, continue through the different supplements, testing which one will correct the situation.

Another concern is a lack of control of the bladder. The loss of ability to control urine flow is often caused by an internal sphincter, and/or external sphincter. (Females have an external orifice). The internal sphincter is an involuntary muscle, while the external sphincter or orifice is voluntarily controlled. Muscles, and/or nerve innervation, can negatively affect urine flow control.

"Is this lack of control being caused by the internal sphincter? external sphincter(orifice)? muscles? nerve innervation?"

There can be more than one reason, so continue testing until there are no other reasons for the incontinence.

This is the conclusion of the urinary system. You now have the knowledge to correct urinary symptoms with this easy-to-use program. Just use it. Trust it. The more you use it, the healthier you will stay.

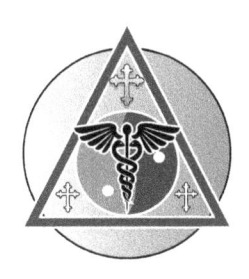

CHAPTER SIXTEEN

The Cause of Disease

There is only one reason for disease – stress. All disease is dis-ease. The body is forced out-of-balance (homeostasis). What causes the stress to start with? That is the million-dollar question answered in this chapter.

The major disruptors of homeostasis, at the physical level, are toxins, parasites, nutritional deficiencies, and/or tissue damage. Although I don't intentionally disregard the other three levels of healing – emotional, mental and spiritual, the majority of this book is devoted to the physical side of healing. For more information on the *Emotional Release Therapy* program refer to Chapter Seventeen. To study the mental and spiritual aspects of the Body Balance Healing System, refer to <u>Resurrecting Your Life</u> by Dr. Jerry Weber.

The content of this chapter is what separates the Body Balance Healing System from conventional medicine and many alternative, natural health practitioners. The difference is knowing how to find the "root cause". That is what everybody desires to know. What is causing it? With the internet at our fingertips, we're getting smarter about our health. We will no longer allow a symptom to be covered up with a medication. We demand answers, and muscle testing can do just that.

Toxins

We live in a toxic world. Babies inherit hundreds of toxins at birth. All of us are bombarded by toxins every day. What are toxins? Toxins are any unnatural substance that is not usable, or bioavailable by the body. It is any substance that creates an imbalance of body function, and places stress on tissue in the body.

There are thousands of toxins in our environment, and more being added every year. These disease causing substances enter the body through the skin, food, air and water. The liver is the hero that deals with detoxing all the toxins that enter the body. Its main purpose is to keep toxins out of the blood so they don't have the chance to run rampant through the body. The liver either disposes a toxin through the bile, or stores it in tissue, keeping it away from vital organs and glands in the body. Over years toxins build up until the "cup runneth over" and symptoms start. A good way to control the amount of toxins that enter your body is to live a clean lifestyle, and take care of the liver. If you take care of your liver, it will take care of you.

Another wonderful tool to cleanse the body of toxins is an infra-red sauna. Safer than the old-fashioned saunas that could get dangerously hot, these saunas heat up to 150 degrees. The main goal of a sauna is to make the body sweat. Sweating is the best way to remove toxins from the body.

There are many different detoxifying techniques, and most of them are effective. Be careful not to detox too much, or too fast. Also, be sure that your elimination systems, including your lymph, and kidneys can detox sufficiently. To make sure ask;

"Can the lymph system eliminate all toxins?"

"Is the liver detoxing all toxins perfectly?"

"Is the blood free of all toxins?"

There should never be toxins in the blood. If there are toxins in the blood, the liver detoxification pathways are not keeping toxins out of the blood, and/or the nephrons in the kidneys are not filtering toxins perfectly. To find out ask;

"Are the liver detoxification pathways keeping all toxins out of the blood?"

"Are the nephrons in the kidneys filtering all toxins out of the blood perfectly?"

The most common symptoms of having toxins in the blood are skin rashes, acne, joint pain, allergies and/or edema. In Chinese medicine, the skin is referred to as the "third kidney." Whenever the kidneys are not functioning perfectly, or are being overwhelmed by an under functioning liver, the skin will show the symptom.

There are too many toxins to name them all. The toxicity chart in the Appendix names the most common toxins, and how to remove them naturally. If the cause of the symptom is a toxin refer to the alphabetical toxin chart.

Parasites

For some people just the word "parasite" makes their skin crawl. I've studied parasites for years and know they are a major contributor to ill health. What are parasites? When I use the term "parasite" I'm not just referring to a worm. The definition that the Body Balance Healing System uses is "any living organism that is using the body as a host."

There are three groups of parasites. 1) Parasitic animals are tapeworms, flukes, round worms, pinworms and protozoa. 2) Micro parasites are pathological bacteria, virus, strep, h pylori bacteria, borrelia burgdorferi (Lyme), babesia, bartonella and chlamydia. 3) Parasitic plants include fungus, mold, black mold, mildew, albicans yeast and microzymas.

Most conventional medical doctors don't believe parasites cause many health issues. But, I know better. I see illnesses, caused by parasites, every day. An infectious agent, or pathogen, is much more common than most medical doctors will admit. They still believe you must leave the United States to catch parasites. This might be true if it is an exotic type of parasite, but not the ones that we positively test for in many patients.

Parasites cause diarrhea, nausea, fatigue, inflammation and pain. All types create waste in the body, which is more harmful to the body than the actual parasite. They also cause nutritional deficiencies by robbing the body of its nutrients, and can cause tissue damage.

Animal parasites are the hardest to kill because these living organisms lay eggs and have a life cycle. You must repeat the same protocol one month after finishing the first protocol to stop the cycle from continuing.

Virus such as Epstein Barr virus, borrelia burgdorferi, shingles virus, and herpes can remain in the body for years, tiring the immune system. These viruses hide inside the cell where they can't be killed. To truly understand these viruses, I suggest reading Medical Medium's book, <u>Mystery Illness</u>. Chapter three explains this concept of virus the best.

Parasitic plants are the entire fungal group, which includes fungus, mold, black mold, mildew, albicans (candida) yeast, and microzymas, to name a few of the most common.

Once it is established that parasites are the main cause, the next step is to test which category the parasite belongs. . .

"Is it a parasitic animal? micro-parasite? parasitic plant?"

The answer should fit in one of the three categories. Once the group is confirmed, refer to the parasitic chart in the Appendix. Muscle test each selection in that category. For instance, if the category is parasitic plant, go to that group on the parasitic chart. Starting with the first choice continue until you get your answer.

"Is the root cause of this health issue fungus? mold? black mold? mildew? albicans yeast? microzymas?"

When the arm or fingers stay strong, signaling a true answer, you have found your problem. Once that parasite is killed, test to see if there are any other parasites causing any of the symptoms. If there is another parasite, begin again at the beginning to find out what type of parasite it is this time. Don't assume that once you kill one parasite that is all. Continue testing until there are no other parasites causing any of the symptoms.

If you are suffering from parasitic activity understand that your body's inner terrain is too acidic. When you are too acidic you will be parasitic and when you are parasitic you are too acidic. When the body is acidic, the macro minerals - calcium, magnesium, potassium and sodium are deficient.

Nutrient Deficiency

Every cell of your body has to receive an abundance of amino acids, vitamins, enzymes, minerals, essential fats, and water. If even one of these substrates are deficient the body slowly begins a deterioration referred to as aging and disease. The challenge today in our fast paced lifestyles and deficient foods it is harder to receive all the nutrients a body needs to operate at optimal function.

The conventional medical community is not concerned about nutrition. Most doctors have had very little training on nutrition. They have been trained to be the professional pill pushers never thinking about why it was happening or how to get the body healthy. Their model is to attack the intruder like they were in war with the body.

Your body has an innate ability to heal naturally. It has the intelligence of running your body every moment of your life. It knows what to do if we give it what it needs and not put stuff in the body that would hurt its ability to heal. One of the most important things is it needs is ample nutrition that can be used by the cell.

Remember - You are no healthier than you are at the cell level. If the food or supplement can not be received and used at the cell level it is not good for the body.

Besides eating a healthy, organic diet every person needs additional supplementation. There are many choices in choosing nutritional products. There is also a major difference in the quality of products. Many of the supplements in drug and grocery stores are synthetic products. Your body is organic tissue and can't use artificial or synthetic substances. When a person buys these types of highly advertised supplements it is a waste of money. Not only can the body not use the supplement, so the body is now deficient in those particular nutrients, but now the body has a harmful toxin to have to deal with and eliminate.

Nutrients are to your body like gas is to your car. You wouldn't think about putting bad gas in your gas tank. Using professional grade supplement will pay off in the long run. They will cost more. Quality does cost, but your body is the only vehicle you will own in this lifetime. All of us have the choice to either pay a little more now for better health or pay the big amounts later in our lives.

Blood tests are only going to show what the amount of nutrients are in the blood. They do not reflect what is happening at the tissue or cell level. Blood tests are helpful but not the full picture as much as people believe. Muscle testing is the perfect tool to test the tissue and cell nutrient levels. You can do this with any tissue, cell or organ.

"Are all amino acids perfect in (whatever tissue, organ, gland or cell you choose)?

If you want to get more specific you could muscle test each individual amino acid. Continue testing each of the different categories of nutrients in the same fashion. Again, in whatever category is not perfect each category can be more specific such as if vitamins were not perfect you could ask;

"Are the water soluble vitamins perfect?"

If they are not, ask;

"Is Vitamin C ? citrus bioflavonoids? B1? B2? B3? B5? B6? B9? B12?"

Test each nutrient in that category. There can be only one in that group but all of them could be deficient. Once that group of vitamins are completed ask;

"Are all fat soluble vitamins perfect?"

If no, ask;

"Is vitamin A? D? E? K? F?"

Do the same with each category. Refer to the nutritional chart in the Appendix for more nutritional choices.

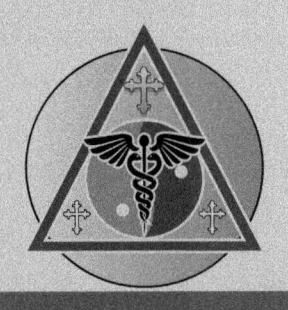

LEVEL 3

ADVANCED

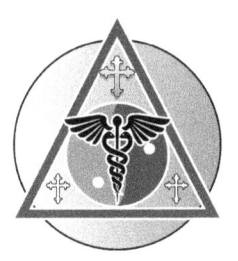

CHAPTER SEVENTEEN
Emotional Release Therapy

Although *You Can Heal – Naturally* is focused on physical aspects of healing it would not be complete without discussing emotions. Most integrative medical doctors and natural health practitioners agree that suppressed emotions play a big part in every dis-ease including cancer.

Emotions are "energy in motion." They are subtle energy that are either positive, empowering emotions such as love, trust, joy, forgiveness and compassion or negative, disempowering emotions such as hate, fear, guilt and envy. Positive emotions flow through the body effortlessly increasing the life force energy which creates vitality and vibrant health. Negative emotions get "stuck" in organs, glands, meridians and chakras which disrupt the natural flow, which causes the life force to be stagnate. Once this starts happening a symptom starts to appear. If these repressed emotions are not found and removed the body can never completely heal.

Once you are a competent muscle tester it is easy to find trapped emotions in the body. The two systems that I personally use are The Emotion Code by Dr. Bradley Nelson and the Emotional Release Therapy, which is taught in this book. Both are good and have their benefits and drawbacks. Anybody who wants to learn about the emotion component of healing should learn both.

I was attending a class that The Emotion Code was being taught. The instructor did an excellent job of teaching the textbook procedures of finding the particular emotion on the chart and how to "swipe" and remove it. She was a certified Emotion Code practitioner and it showed. At the end of the class the instructor asked if there were any questions. I raised my hand and asked a shocking question: would you like to know how to release emotions much faster? Of course, she was surprised to hear such a claim and asked me to show the class.

I asked for a volunteer from the audience who felt like they had trapped emotions. Through muscle testing I demonstrated that her heart had over fifty trapped emotions. I explained that if I used The Emotion Code each separate emotion would have to be selected from the chart and three swipes for each trapped emotion would have to be performed. It was easy to calculate the process would take a minimum of 150 swipes.

I explained that using the Emotional Release Therapy it would only take 15 swipes to remove all of them! The class couldn't believe it. How could that possibly work? The only way to prove my point was to do it. After only fifteen swipes and the "five magic words" I demonstrated that the lady's heart was now "happy" and no trapped emotions remained.

I learned about the importance of "trapped emotions" from Dr. Nelson. He is the "father" of the current emotional release programs. The Emotion Code taught me how to find these negative blocks of energy and eliminate them. I am very grateful Dr. Brad showed all of us how this part of healing works. He has personally stated there is more to discover about dealing with repressed emotions. The Emotional Release Therapy program provides more of that information that I have found by using his information and building on it.

The biggest advantage of the Emotional Release Therapy is speed. I am not a certified Emotion Code practitioner. I am a busy naturopath doctor who understands the importance of removing these toxic emotions. By using this system, I can quickly remove these roadblocks to better health and move on to the physical issues causing the symptom. In most cases there is no need to talk about these repressed feelings and move on.

Some people might want to pick out each emotion and talk about it. If that is true, The Emotion Code is the perfect tool. If you just want to remove as many as possible as fast as you can then the Emotional Release Therapy is the better choice. Sometimes after doing the Emotional Release

Therapy some emotions do not get released. Inherited emotions or trapped emotions that did not get released require using The Emotion Code.

Think of a room that is dark (low energy, negative, trapped emotions). What happens when the light is turned on? As we all know, the darkness disappears. Where did the darkness go? Did it leave? Of course not. It was transformed into a higher vibration by the highest frequency of light. As the Bible says, "let there be light."

Trapped, repressed emotions are low energy and dark. Positive, Godly emotions such as love, trust, forgiveness, gratitude and peace are some of the highest vibrations. These words change the darkness into light. They neutralize the darkness by changing the darkness into light and healing.

The Emotional Release Therapy Techniques

The first step of doing an emotional release is to know how to find where the trapped emotions are located. Every organ, gland, chakra or meridian can have trapped emotions. The easiest technique of finding a repressed emotion is to ask;

"Is this organ, gland, chakra or meridian happy?"

If an area is not "happy" it has at least one and possibly many trapped emotions. These trapped emotions can be conscious and/or subconscious. Conscious trapped emotions will answer directly when it is asked if it is "happy". But the subconscious does not answer the same way.

To find subconscious emotions do the "thymus point." Use the pointer finger and the middle finger, which is positive and negative charge, and point directly at the thymus gland. You can easily find subconscious trapped emotions, simply by naming the organ, gland, chakra or meridian while doing the thymus point. Anything that tests weak has subconscious trapped emotions. You can also ask;

"Is this organ, gland, chakra or meridian happy subconsciously?"

I believe the thymus point is easier but either one will work. You don't have to do both. Make sure not to lay your finger down against the thymus. It is an actual pointing like writing with a pencil. This should not be confused with the thymus thump taught by Donna Eden.

Once the conscious or subconscious trapped emotions are located it is time to remove them. The first thing to do is to count how many trapped emotions there are in the selected area. If there are under five The Emotion Code is best. If the total is more than five, then the Emotional Release Therapy program is a better choice.

There are two basic types of trapped emotions – personal and inherited. This is true for both conscious and subconscious. If there are over five personal trapped emotions use the Emotional Release Therapy program. To find out ask;

"How many trapped emotions are in this organ, gland, chakra or meridian?"
"Are all of these personal trapped emotions?"

You now know how many trapped emotions there are in this tissue. By asking the second question you know what percentage of these trapped emotions are personal or inherited. If there are over five personal trapped emotions use the Emotional Release Therapy program. If it is under five or inherited use The Emotion Code.

To remove trapped emotions requires using the "swiping technique" which is taught in both programs. Using the palm of your hand or a magnet start at the bridge of the nose and move up over the middle of the head to the nape. This movement traces the governing meridian.

The "Five Magic Words" are used in conjunction with "swiping" to change the vibration and remove the lower energy. These five words are **Love**; **Trust**; **Forgiveness**; **Gratitude**; and **Peace**. By doing three swipes per word while placing your intention and focus toward the organ, gland, chakra or meridian will remove the trapped emotions. If the trapped emotions are subconscious your eyes should be closed while swiping. If the trapped emotions are conscious the eyes should be open. Intention is very important. Energy follows thought. Also breathing into the affected area while swiping is beneficial.

Once these fifteen well-intentioned swipes are completed double check to make sure all trapped emotions have been cleared by asking;

"Is this organ, gland, chakra or meridian happy consciously and subconsciously (or use the thymus point while asking the same question the second time).

If the answer is yes for both conscious and subconscious this area is free of trapped emotions. You are ready to locate the next area that has trapped emotions. If the answer is no refer to The Emotion Code and pick out what emotions did not get removed. In my experience the Emotional Release Therapy program removes almost all personal trapped emotions.

At one class we performed a group emotional release. Knowing that the heart controls the emotional condition of the body I directed the class to muscle test if their heart was happy. Out of the thirty students most had hearts that were not happy, meaning there were trapped emotions. Next, together we did the Emotional Release program and everybody's heart in the group changed to the perfect vibration of 540 (David Hawkins Map of Consciousness) except for one lady. At that time, we referred to The Emotion Code chart and found that there were two trapped emotions – abandonment and betrayal. As soon as we pointed out the two emotions the lady admitted that her husband was cheating on her.

By these two emotions not releasing gave her the opportunity to talk about it and get it off her chest. Sometimes the person needs to talk about their emotions. If that is the case the body will not remove the trapped emotion. When the Emotional Release Therapy removes all of the trapped emotions you know there are none that need to be verbalized. At this time you are done with the exam and this chapter.

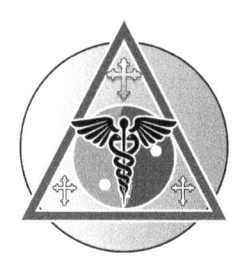

CHAPTER EIGHTEEN

It's All About Frequency – The Secret

"If you want to find the secrets of the universe (body) think in terms of energy, frequency and vibration."

Nikola Tesla

Albert Einstein stated, "Everything in life is vibration." Everything in the universe is moving. When something moves it creates a vibration, which can be measured by frequency. Frequency is a logarithm which can be measured, and logged with a particular number. Frequency is measured scientifically in Hz (hertz). In the Body Balance Healing System logarithm numbers are used, not based from Hz. These numbers have been carefully tested through muscle testing to be perfectly accurate.

Every atom of every cell in the body is moving. When the body resonates at the perfect vibration it is healthy, and vibrant. The body is free of symptoms, and illness, as long as the body's vibrations stay high. Every negative thought, toxin, nutritional deficiency or trapped emotion will lower this "healthy" vibration. It will no longer oscillate at the perfect vibration. This slower, lower vibration causes dis-ease and imbalance of homeostasis (balance) in the body. Over time this creates symptoms, and eventually disease.

Each of us have our own "personal vibration" which dictates the condition of our health. The "healthy" vibration, that we are born with, decreases as we age because of the years of accumulation of negative thoughts, fears, disempowering beliefs, toxins, parasites, nutritional deficiencies and tissue damage. This lower energy is blamed on aging, but the real culprit is the buildup of toxic waste, both physically, emotionally and mentally.

Every negative, fearful thought or action lowers your vibration and every higher, positive, Godly thought or action raises your vibration. Higher vibration creates better health. Lower vibration brings on illness. With this concept in mind, it's possible to change the condition of any illness or disease, simply by being more aware of our thoughts and actions, and changing what is not bringing us joy, happiness and health. For more information on this important step in your healing journey refer to my book <u>Resurrecting Your Life.</u>

The Finger Print Frequency System

The Finger Print Frequency System can measure the "personal vibration" of any tissue, cell, organ or gland. It enables you to find the exact frequency of each toxin, parasite and/or nutritional deficiency that is causing the lower vibration. The recorded frequencies in this book are as accurate as the FBI finger prints of a person. This advanced technique is faster and more specific than the basic four causes of disease. Once you learn how to use this system you will never go back to the basic four causes.

I was introduced to the concept of using frequency by my mentor, Dr. James Overmann. I remember him explaining to me two frequency numbers. He explained to me that $12.9\text{-}15$ (twelve nine to the fifteenth power) was perfect health. Below 12.9 (twelve nine) was the frequency of parasitic activity. When I was introduced to this secret of health, I didn't see the importance. I already knew how to find the root cause by using the four causes so I questioned why I needed to understand frequency.

It took years for me to clearly see the importance of learning frequencies. Once I understood the power of muscle testing frequencies, I started using muscle testing to calculate and log frequency numbers for every toxin, parasite and nutrient that I discovered. Today, I use frequencies to find the root cause on 100% of our patients. Here is how the Finger Print Frequency System is used;

12.9-15 is the frequency of perfect health in all tissue in the body and brain. I was teaching a seminar for forty natural health professionals and I started the program by announcing I was going to share with them what "perfect health" was. There were many skeptical looks as I made my claim. I asked a lady from the audience if I could muscle test her to prove my point. I showed the audience how muscle testing worked.

After establishing a true/false baseline that the audience was comfortable with, I was ready to prove my point. As the practitioners watched, I demonstrated how the arm reacted weak when I made the statement "perfect health is 12.9-14.99999 or lower." Then I tested again, changing the statement to "perfect health is 12.9-15.00001 or higher. Both times the arm could not resist my pressure. But, when I made the statement that "perfect health is exactly 12.9-15" the muscle tested strong, representing a true answer.

> *"Our entire biological system – the brain and the earth itself work on the same frequencies."*
>
> *Nikola Tesla*

This one frequency can quickly tell you what organ, gland or vessel is not functioning perfectly. To vibrate at this frequency the selected tissue must be functioning perfectly, free of all toxins, parasites, tissue damage and nutritional deficiencies. To use this "frequency" check just ask;

"Is this organ, gland, system, tissue, or cell frequency exactly "twelve – nine to the fifteenth power?"

If it is not vibrating at this frequency use the frequency cascade, and ask;

"Is this tissue vibrating over 12.9-15?"

Since you have already designated that the tissue is not vibrating at the perfect frequency, it is either under, or over the perfect frequency. If the above test stays strong, refer to the frequencies on the toxicity charts above 12.9-15. If the question tests false, you look at the charts for the frequency numbers under 12.9-15. The toxicity, parasite and nutritional charts in the Appendix will guide you to the specific frequency which gives you the root cause.

If the cause is over 12.9-15 you will start your search in the toxicity chart. This is the only chart that will have frequencies over 12.9-15. Test which section of the chart the root cause is located by asking;

"Is the root cause above 12.9-100? 12.9-200? 12.9-1000? 12.9-2000?

If the root cause is above 12.9-15, but below 12.9-100, test each toxin listed in that category. If the root cause is above 12.9-100, but not above 12.9-200, test the toxins in that category. Continue this elimination process until you find the range of frequency, and refer to that part of the chart.

Once you find the exact toxin, the chart will give you the specific frequency for that particular toxin. It also shows you the "relative compatibility" of that toxin and the supplement that is recommended to remove it.

Every illness, including cancer, is a frequency that is not the perfect vibration. If you are experiencing pain, or any symptom, the particular tissue is not 12.9-15. The muscle tester's job is to determine if it is above or below the perfect frequency. This can be accomplished very easily once you are confident of muscle testing.

Testing by frequency is an advanced technique that I don't recommend for beginning muscle testers. This is why we have included both toxicity charts -one in alphabetical order and the other chart that where the toxins are ranked by frequency, Both can be used for crosschecking.

Using a frequency check after you have the tissue functioning at 100% is ideal because tissue can function at 100% and not be the perfect frequency. If the frequency is not perfect, but functioning is 100%, usually denotes a nutritional deficiency that is not affecting the functioning of that tissue, but is not perfect.

Relative Compatibility

What is relative compatibility? This concept came to me when I asked the question, "why is this toxin or parasite in this particular tissue?" Why did it "pick" that certain organ? As the Bible promises – ask and you shall find. What I found is called "relative compatibility."

The Law of Attraction states that "like attracts like." Relative compatibility is a magnetic, energetic attraction in tissue caused by a nutritional deficiency. Each different nutritional deficiency sends out a unique SOS signal. There is one particular toxin or parasite, if available in the body, "answers" the call for help, entering that tissue. But, instead of helping the tissue, the toxin or parasite causes more imbalance and disfunction.

These "helpers" actually are like terrorists attacking a weak country. If the tissue is strong these "invaders" can't penetrate the borders. But, as soon as one nutrient is not sufficient (below 95%), it opens the door for the toxin or parasite to enter.

The deficiency of the nutrient(s) always happen first, before the toxin or parasite enters. This can be proven via muscle testing. When a system is not functioning sufficiently, there has to be an organ or gland in that system not working sufficiently. This means there is either tissue or cells not functioning sufficiently in the particular organ or gland. Why is it not functioning at least sufficiently? The root cause is one or more of the four causes discussed earlier. Once you test which of the four reasons is the primary root cause ask;

"Is there a reason why this toxin or parasite is in this tissue or cell?"

If the answer is "yes", ask;

"Is it a mineral deficiency? amino acid deficiency? vitamin deficiency? essential fatty acid deficiency?"

Use the nutritional grid chart in the Appendix to select the missing nutrient(s). Once the nutrient deficiency is decided, ask;

"Can this nutrient be utilized perfectly in this tissue?"

If "yes", add that nutrient to your daily regimen. If "no", find out why it can't be utilized;

"Can this nutrient be digested sufficiently? absorbed through the GI tract sufficiently? metabolized sufficiently? Are the nutrient receptors at the cell level working sufficiently?"

If you receive a "no" on any of these questions, go back and use the system to find the cause and repair the imbalance.

Sometimes there will not be a reason why the toxin or parasite is in the tissue. It will seem like the concept is untrue, but it's not, and can be verified by muscle testing, Ask;

"Was there a nutrient deficiency in this tissue before the toxin or parasite?"

The answer will be "yes" – every time. Many times, the toxin or parasite has been in the tissue for a long time, sometimes years. Over that span of time the nutrient deficiency has been corrected.

If a parasite is in the tissue a trace mineral deficiency is the nutritional deficiency, but a weak immune system for that particular tissue can also be the cause. Sometimes it can be both. The immune system that controls this area will be functioning under 50%. This is like the army not strong enough to keep the invaders out. If there is a parasite in the tissue you need to test to see if the parasite can be killed at this time. If it can't be killed at this time it is usually because of a weak immune system. Refer to the chapter on the immune system.

Sometimes the parasite can be killed immediately but other times you have to repair the immune system first before the parasite can be killed. To find out ask;

"Can this parasite be killed at this time?"

If "yes", refer to the parasite chart, establish the type of parasite and what supplement will kill it. If "no," ask why.

"Is it because of the immune system?"

It usually will be the immune system. The practice of using a supplement to boost the entire immune system is good, but not specific enough. Every organ or gland has a specific part of the immune system that is responsible for their immune system function. To find the location where the immune system is weak just ask;

"Is this weak immune system caused by the white pulp of the spleen? GALT? thymus? bone marrow?"

The answer will be in one of these areas where the tissue will usually be functioning under 50%. By correcting the immune system will allow the parasite to be killed and make the body's defenses stronger.

Relative Compatibility is a step above just finding the root cause, and correcting the imbalance. By using the concept of Relative Compatibility, weak tissue will be rebuilt, creating a stronger, healthier body. Discovering not only the root cause, but the "why" of the root cause, the nutrient deficiency causing the weakness will be corrected.

These two unique concepts can help even the most advanced practitioner improve their results. Using the Finger Print Frequency System, you can quickly determine the root cause. By testing with frequencies, instead of functioning, is another advanced method of muscle testing.

You have now been given information that very few people know. It is new, exciting and it works. These two new techniques will take your muscle testing skills to a new level of excellence and produce better results for you, your family, friends, clients and patients. With all the information in the last eighteen chapters, you now are ready for the answers. The Appendix is a collection of charts which you will use on your health quest. Enjoy the journey and keep on muscle testing. The more you muscle test, the better muscle tester you will become. Using the techniques and knowledge in *You Can Heal - Naturally* can help you become a master muscle tester.

"Muscle test a (wo)man and you balance him/her for a day. Teach a (wo)man to muscle test and you balance him or her for life."

Touch For Health Proverb

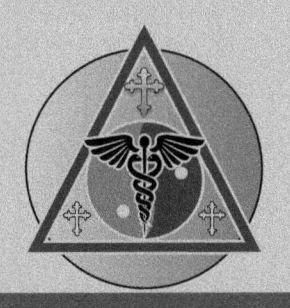

APPENDIX

APPENDIX – LIST OF CONTENTS

1. The 5 Steps to Better Health

2. The Body Balance Healing System Assessment Form

3. Nutritional Deficiency Chart

4. Key for Supplement Companies Used in the Charts

5. Nutritional Supplement Chart

6. Toxin Charts (Alphabetical)

7. Parasite Charts (Parasitic Animals, Parasitic Plants, Micro-Parasites, Parasites)

8. Frequency Cascade Chart

9. Digestion Chart

10. Tissue Damage

11. Toxin Charts (by Frequency)

12. Contact Information

THE 5 STEPS TO BETTER HEALTH

1. <u>Select</u> one of the ten systems where the root cause is located.

2. <u>Locate</u> the precise part of that system where the imbalance is.

3. <u>Measure</u> the functioning of the area that is testing as the root cause.

4. <u>Determine</u> the reason why it is not functioning perfectly.

5. <u>Choose</u> which supplement is best to correct the imbalance.

Body Balance Healing System — Assessment Form

Name _____ Date of Birth _____ Date _____ Follow Up _____
(First and Last)

1. Circulatory: ____ Blood: ____ Blood Flow: ____ Viscosity: ____ Heart: ____ Arteries: ____ Veins: ____ Capillaries: ____

2. Digestive: ____ Protein Digestion: ____ Fat Digestion: ____ Sugar Digestion: ____ Starch Digestion: ____ Salivary glands: ____ Esophagus: ____ Lower Esophageal Valve: ____ Stomach: ____ Liver: ____ Gallbladder: ____ Bile Duct: ____ Bile Salts: ____

3. Intestinal: ____ Duodenum: ____ Jejunum: ____ Villi: ____ Microvilli: ____ Ileum: ____ Ileocecal Valve: ____ Cecum: ____ Ascending Colon: ____ Hepatic Flexur: ____ Tranverse Colon: ____ Splenic Flexor: ____ Descending Colon: ____ Sigmoid Colon: ____ Rectum: ____ Anus: ____

4. Glandular: ____ Adrenal: ____ Hypothalamus: ____ Pancreas: ____ Pituitary: ____ Pineal: ____ Spleen: ____ Thyroid: ____ Parathyroid: ____

5. Immune: ____ Tonsils: ____ Lymph Glands: ____ Lymph Nodes: ____ Lymph Ducts: ____ Thymus: ____ Bone Marrow: ____ Cysterna Chyli: ____ Lymph Fluid: ____ Spleen: ____

6. Nervous: ____ Brain: ____ Cranial N: ____ Spinal Cord: ____ Spinal Nerves: ____ Parasympathetic: ____ Sympathetic: ____ Sensory N: ____ Motor N: ____ Cutaneous N: ____ Nerve Receptors: ____

7. Reproductive: ____
   - Male: ____ Testes: ____ Prostate: ____ Hormones: ____ Penis: ____
   - Female: ____ Ovaries: ____ Uterus: ____ Hormones: ____ Cervix: ____ Fallopian Tubes: ____ Vagina: ____

8. Respiratory: ____ Paranasal (Upper) Sinus: ____ Bronchiols: ____ Lungs: ____ Diaphragm: ____ Phrenic N: ____

9. Structural: ____ Bones: ____ Joints: ____ Muscles: ____ Skin: ____ Connective Tissue: ____ Fascia: ____ Soft Tissue: ____

10. Urinary: ____ Kidney: ____ Nephrons: ____ Ureters: ____ Bladder: ____ Internal Urethral Sphincter: ____ External Urethral Sphincter (M) Orifice (f): ____ Urethra: ____

Reasons for Symptoms:

1. Parasite ____   3. Nutritional Deficiency ____   5. Emotional ____
2. Toxin ____   4. Tissue Damage ____

Symptom	Recommendations
#1 Symptom _____	_____
#2 Symptom _____	_____
#3 Symptom _____	_____
#4 Symptom _____	_____

Nutritional Deficiency Chart

ROW		A	B	C
1	1.1	Acidophilus	Gold	Protein
	1.2	Amino Acid	Indium	Pyridoxine (B6)
	1.3	Antimony	Iodine	Rhodium
	1.4	Barium	Iron	Riboflavin (B2)
2	2.1	Beta Carotene	Lanthanum	Selenium
	2.2	Bile Salts	Lecithin	Silica
	2.3	Bioflavonoids	Lithium	Sodium
	2.4	Bismuth	Magnesium	Strontium
3	3.1	Boron	Manganese	Sulfur
	3.2	Bromine	Molybdenum	Thallium
	3.3	Calcium	Niacin (B3)	Thiamine (B1)
	3.4	Cell Salts	Nickle	Trace Mineral
4	4.1	Chloride	Nitric Oxide	Vanadium
	4.2	Chromium	Omega 3	Vitamin A
	4.3	Co-Q 10	Omega 6	Vitamin B
	4.4	Cobalt	Palladium	Vitamin C
5	5.1	Copper	Pantothenic Acid (B5)	Vitamin D
	5.2	Cyanocobalamin (B12)	Phosphorus	Vitamin E
	5.3	Folate (B9)	Platinum	Vitamin F
	5.4	Germanium	Potassium	Zinc

*Key for Supplement Companies Used in the Charts

Abbreviation	Name of Company	Abbreviation	Name of Company
BR	Biotics Research	P	Perque
DL	Douglas Labs	PE	Pure Encapsulation
H&W	Health & Wellness of Carmel	RN	Researched Nutritionals
L	Loomis Enzymes	TH	Thorne
M	Metagenics	W	Wellgenix
N	XYMOG	Z	Zorex
NM	NutraMedix		

Nutritional Supplement Chart*

ROW		A	B	C
1	1.1	ION Gut Health (ION) Bio-Dolph-7 Plus (BR)	Sea Essentials (W)	IvD (L)
	1.2	IvD (L), Amino Acid Quick-Sorb (BR), Perfect Amino (Body Health)	Sea Essentials (W) Multi-Mins (BR) Iodizyme-HP (B)	B6/B1 (Z) Pyridoxal-5'-Phosphate (Th)
	1.3	Sea Essentials (W) Multi-Mins (BR)	Liquid Iodine Forte (BR) KI Caps (Z)	Sea Essentials (W) BioDrive (BR)
	1.4	Sea Essentials (W)	Iron (H&W)	Riboflavin Complex (Z) Bio-GGG-B (BR)
2	2.1	Bio-Ae-Mulsion (BR)	Sea Essentials (W)	Se-Zyme Forte (BR) Sea Essentials (W)
	2.2	Digestamax (H&W)	Phosphatidylcholine (BR) BIL (L) Phosphatidylserine (H&W)	Sea Essentials (W) Multi-Mins (BR)
	2.3	OPT (L) AHF (BR)	Li-Zyme (BR) Lithium (PE)	ADB5-Plus (BR)
	2.4	Sea Essentials (W) Pyloricil (PE)	OptiMag (H&W) Multi-Mins (BR)	Sea Essentials (W) Strontium Citrate (PE) Strontium Citrate (Z)
3	3.1	Sea Essentials (W) Boron (Z), Multi-Mins (BR)	Sea Essentials (W) Manganese (PE) Multi-Mins (BR)	MSM Plus (Z) Multi-Mins (BR)
	3.2	Sea Essentials (W)	Molybdenum (DL) Multi-Mins (BR)	Sea Essentials (W) Multi-Mins (BR)
	3.3	Bio-CMP (BR), CLM (L) Multi-Mins (BR)	Niacin 100 (BR) Niacin non-flush (H&W)	B-Complex (BR) B6/B1 (Z)
	3.4	Bioplasma Cell Salts (Hyland's)	Sea Essentials (W) Multi-Mins (BR)	Sea Essentials (W) Multi-Mins (BR)

ROW		A	B	C
4	4.1	Sea Essentials (W) ASEA (Redox) Multi-Mins (BR)	Nitric Oxide MAX (H&W) Arginine Complex (Z)	Sea Essentials (W) Bio-Multi Plus (BR) GlucoBalance (BR)
	4.2	Chromium (H&W) Cr-Zyme (BR) Multi-Mins (BR)	Optimal EFA (H&W) Omega III (H&W)	Bio-AE-Mulsion (BR)
	4.3	CoQ-10 (H&W) CoQ-Zyme 100 Plus (BR)	Sun Flax (Z)	B-Complex (BR) B Complex (H&W)
	4.4	Sea Essentials (W) Multi-Mins (BR)	Sea Essentials (W)	Opt (L) Ascorbic Acid (PE), AHF (BR)
5	5.1	Sea Essentials (W) Cu-Zyme (BR) Multi-Mins (BR)	Pantethine (Th) B Complex (Z)	Bio-D-Mulsion (BR) K2&D (H&W)
	5.2	Methyl B12 Plus (DL) Activated B-12 Guard (Perque) both sublingual	Super Phosphozyme (BR) Bone Builder (Metagenics)	Mixed E (H&W)
	5.3	L-Methylfolate	Sea Essentials (W)	Omega III (H&W) Flax Seed Oil
	5.4	Sea Essentials (W)	Bio-CMP (BR), Potassium HP (BR), Multi-Mins (BR)	Zn-Zyme (BR) Zinc Chelate (H&W)

Toxin Chart (Alphabetical)

Toxin	Frequency	Deficiency	Supplement/Company*
Aflatoxins	12.9^{1999}	Vitamin C	ENV/GBLV Homeopathic (Z)
Asbestos	$12.9^{89.7}$	Calcium	ENV/GBLV Homeopathic (Z)
Aspartame	12.9^{199}	Omega3	ENV/GBLV Homeopathic (Z)
Candida Toxins	$12.9^{14.69}$	Trace Minerals	Candida Homeopathic (Z)
DDT	12.9^{79}	Trace Mineral	Beta Plus (BR)
Dioxin	$12.9^{89.9}$	Magnesium	ENV/GBLV Homeopathic (Z)
Environmental	$12.9^{14.68}$	B^2 (riboflavin)	ENV/GBLV Homeopathic (Z)
Formaldehyde	12.9^{2099}	Vitamin C	ENV/GBLV Homeopathic (Z)
Glyphosate	12.9^{1003}	Tissue Cell Salts	L-Lysine HCL (BR)
GMO	12.9^{99}	Phosphorus	Bromelain Plus CLA (BR)
Heavy Metal (each HMT has slightly different frequency)	$12.9^{14.53}$	Trace Mineral	Porphyra-Zyme (BR) Chelex (XYMOGEN)
Herbicides	12.9^{198}	Calcium/ Magnesium	L-Lysine HCL (BR)
Insecticides	12.9^{2799}	B Complex	GB Complete (Z) Beta Plus (BR)
Ionic HMT	$12.9^{14.798}$	Trace Mineral	GB Complete (Z) Beta Plus (BR)
Mercury/ Aluminum Compound	12.9^{1004}	Trace Mineral	GB Complete (Z)
Metabolic Toxin	$12.9^{14.78}$	B^1 (thiamine)	ENV/GBLV Homeopathic (Z)
Mold Toxins	$12.9^{14.2}$	Vitamin C & Bioflavonoids	Mold Antigen (Z)
MSG	12.9^{2009}	Trace Mineral	ENV/GBLV Homeopathic (Z)
Neurotoxin	$12.9^{14.77}$	Calcium	ENV/GBLV Homeopathic (Z)
Nitrates	12.9^{2599}	Mag/Cal/ Potassium (K) receptors	Dysbiocide (BR)
Organophosphates	$12.9^{14.799}$	Trace Mineral	Beta TCP (BR), 7-Ketozym (BR)
Parabens	12.9^{2199}	Calcium	GSH Plus (BR)
Parasite Toxins	$12.9^{14.57}$	Vitamin C	Para Comp Herbal (Z)

Toxin	Frequency	Deficiency	Supplement/Company*
Pesticides	$12.9^{2899.7}$	Magnesium	Beta Plus (BR)
PCB	$12.9^{14.59}$	Mag/Cal/K/Sodium	Gingko Biloba (BR)
Phthalates	$12.9^{14.1}$	Potassium	GSH Plus (BR)
Plastic	$12.9^{14.39}$	Magnesium	GSH Plus (BR)
Sodium Lauryl Sulfate	12.9^{1899}	Potassium	MSM Plus (Z)
Solvents	$12.9^{14.79}$	Trace Minerals	MSM Plus (Z)
Styrene	$12.9^{14.76}$	Sodium	7-Ketozym (BR)
Sulfates	$12.9^{2899.9}$	Mag/Cal/K receptors	Bio-6-Plus (BR), MSM Plus (Z)
Toxic Gold	12.9^{999}	Vitamin E	Bio-3-BG both (BR)

Parasite Chart

Frequency Range >12.8 and <12.9			
Parasitic Animals			
Name	Deficiency	Emotion*	Supplement/Company*
Amoebae	Molybdenum	Insecurity	Emulsified Organic Oregano, (EOO) Blend (Z), ENULA (NM)
Arthropods	Chromium	Blaming	(EOO) Blend (Z) SAMENTO (NM)
Flukes	Zinc	Dread	(EOO) Blend (Z) CONDURA (NM)
Protozoa	Bromine	Fear	(EOO) Blend (Z), ENULA (NM)
Ringworm	Cerium	Vulnerability	(EOO) Blend (Z), ENULA (NM)
Roundworm	Iodine	Bitterness	(EOO) Blend (Z) BARBERRY (NM)
Tapeworm	Indium	Anger	(EOO) Blend (Z) SAMENTO (NM)
Parasitic Plants			
Name	Deficiency	Emotion*	Supplement/Company*
Black Mold	Indium	Abandonment	Mold Antigen (Z), ADP (BR)
Candida	Thallium	Heartache	Candida (Z)
Fungi	Germanium	Discouragement	CUMANDA (NM)
Microzymas	Vanadium	Betrayal	Pneuma-Zyme (BR)
Mildew	Manganese	Lost	QUINA (NM), CUMANDA (NM)
Mold	Chromium	Forlorn	Mold Antigen (Z), ADP (BR)
Slime Mold	Nickle	Love Unreceived	Mold Antigen (Z), ADP (BR)
Yeasts (Albicans)	Thallium	Heartache	Candida (Z)

| Micro-Parasites ||||
Name	Deficiency	Emotion*	Supplement/Company*
Bacteria (Pathological)	Copper	Anxiety	Complete Kare Spray (Z), BANDEROL (NM)
Borrelia Burgdorferi (Lyme)	Antimony	Despair	Berberine HCL (Z), BANDEROL (NM), TEASAL (NM)
C-Dif	Gold	Helplessness	Microbinate (RN)
E-Coli	Barium	Rejection	ADP (BR)
Epstein Barr Virus	Sulfur	Sadness	Berberine HCL (Z) TAKUNA (NM)
Hepatitis C Virus	Lanthanum	Defensiveness	Viral Homeopathic (Z)
Herpes I	Manganese	Sorrow	BARBERRY (NM)
Herpes II (Genital)	Chloride	Forlorn	QUINA (NM)
H. Pylori Bacteria	Gold	Betrayal	TomKat (Z)
Influenza (Flu)	Rhodium	Sorrow	Flu Homeopathic (Z)
Nanobacteria	Selenium	Insecurity	TomKat (Z)
Salmonella	Selenium	Abandonment	HOUTTUYNIA (NM)
Shingles Virus	Bismuth	Lost	BARBERRY (NM)
Strep	Silica	Betrayal	Microbinate (RN)
Staph	Indium	Anxiety	TAKUNA (NM)
Zoster Virus	Palladium	Effort Unreceived	BARBERRY (NM)

Parasite Chart, continued

Frequency Range >12.9 and <12.9[11]			
Parasites			
Name	Deficiency	Emotion*	Supplement/Company*
Babesia	Aluminum	Failure	BANDEROL (NM)
Bartonella	Iron	Blaming	HOUTTUYNIA (NM)
Chlamydia	Molybdenum	Forlorn	Viral Homeopathic (Z)
Corona Virus	Cobalt	Abandonment	Para Comp (Z)
Ehrlichia	Cesium	Lost	QUINA (NM)
Giardia	Iodine	Effort Unreceived	TomKat (Z)
Human Papilloma Virus	Chloride	Love Unreceived	HOUTTUYNIA (NM)
Mycoplasma	Tin	Rejection	Pneuma-Zyme (BR)

*All emotions taken from *The Emotion Code* by Dr. Bradley Nelson

Frequency Cascade Chart

Frequency	Condition	Use
Above 12.9[15]	Toxins	See Toxin Charts (Frequency)
12.9[15] is PERFECT HEALTH		
12.9[14.9]	Adhesions	Se-Zyme Forte (BR)
12.9[14.8]	Enzyme Deficiency	See Digestion Chart
>12.9[14] and <12.9[14.8]	Toxins	See Toxin Charts (Frequency)
12.9[13]	Nutritional Deficiency	See Nutritional Deficiency Chart
12.9[12]	Pharmaceutical Toxins	Dysbiocide (BR)
12.9[11]	Tissue Damage	See Tissue Damage Chart
>12.9[9] and <12.9[11]	Parasites	See Parasite Chart
12.9 and <12.9[10]	Repressed (Suppressed) Emotions	See Emotional Release Therapy Chart
<12.9	Parasites	See Parasite Chart

Digestion Chart

Type of Digestion	Supplement/Company*
Protein	GastroMax – contains HCl (H&W), TRMA (L), Intenzyme Forte (BR), HCL (L)
Fat	VSCLR (L), Digestamax (L), Bil (L)
Sugar/Carbs	PAN (L), DGST (L)

Tissue Damage

Tissue Type	Supplement/Company*
Circulatory	Circ (L), Cytozyme-H (BR)
Digestive	STM (L), Gastrazyme (BR), Cytozyme-LV (BR)
Intestinal	Gastrazyme (BR), ION Gut Health (ION), IPS (BR)
Glandular	Cytozyme-AD (BR), Cytozyme-PT/HPT (BR), Cytozyme-PAN (BR), Cytozyme-THY (BR), ADR (L), Adrenal Cortex (TH)
Immune	Cytozyme-SP (BR), Cytozyme-THY (BR), Bio-Immunozyme Forte (BR)
Lymph	Circ (L)
Nervous	CLM (L), ADHS (BR), Cytozyme-B (BR), SYM (L), Lithium Orotate (Z)
Reproductive	Fem (L), Mal (L), Cytomzyme-F (BR), Cytozyme-M (BR)
Respiratory	Rsp (L), Pneuma-Zyme (BR), OOrganik 15 (BR)
Structural	Osteo-B Plus (BR), OSTEO (L), NAC (BR), MSCLR (L), Skn (L), TRMA (L), IVD (L), Cytozyme LV (BR)
Urinary	Kdy (L), Renal Plus (BR), Cytomzyme-KD (BR), URT (L)

Toxin Chart (by Frequency)

Frequency Range >12.9^{14} and <12.9$^{14.8}$			
Frequency	Toxin	Deficiency	Supplement/Company*
12.9$^{14.1}$	Phthalates	Potassium	GSH Plus (BR)
12.9$^{14.2}$	Mold Toxins	Vitamin C & Bioflavonoids	Mold Antigen (Z)
12.9$^{14.39}$	Plastic	Magnesium	GSH Plus (BR)
12.9$^{14.53}$	Heavy Metal (each HMT has slightly different frequency)	Trace Mineral	Porphyra-Zyme (BR) or Chelex (XYMOGEN)
12.9$^{14.57}$	Parasite Toxins	Vitamin C	Para Comp Herbal (Z)
12.9$^{14.59}$	PCB	Mag/Cal/ Potassium / Sodium	Gingko Biloba (BR)
12.9$^{14.68}$	Environmental	B2 (riboflavin)	ENV/GBLV Homeopathic (Z)
12.9$^{14.69}$	Candida Toxins	Trace Minerals	Candida Homeopathic (Z)
12.9$^{14.76}$	Styrene	Sodium	7-Ketozym (BR)

$12.9^{14.77}$	Neurotoxin	Calcium	ENV/GBLV Homeopathic (Z)
$12.9^{14.78}$	Metabolic Toxin	B1 (thiamine)	ENV/GBLV Homeopathic (Z)
$12.9^{14.79}$	Solvents	Trace Minerals	MSM Plus (Z)
$12.9^{14.798}$	Ionic HMT	Trace Mineral	GB Complete (Z) Beta Plus (BR)
$12.9^{14.799}$	Organophosphates	Trace Mineral	Beta TCP (BR), 7-Ketozym Forte (BR)

Frequency 12.9^{15} is PERFECT HEALTH

Frequencies Range >12.9^{15} and <12.9^{100}

Frequency	Toxin	Deficiency	Supplement/Company*
12.9^{79}	DDT	Trace Mineral	Beta Plus (BR)
$12.9^{89.7}$	Asbestos	Calcium	ENV/GBLV Homeopathic (Z)
$12.9^{89.9}$	Dioxin	Magnesium	ENV/GBLV Homeopathic (Z)
12.9^{99}	GMO	Phosphorus	Bromelain Plus CLA (BR)

Frequency Range >12.9^{100} and <12.9^{1000}

Frequency	Toxin	Deficiency	Supplement/Company*
12.9^{198}	Herbicides	Calcium/ Magnesium	L-Lysine HCL (BR)
12.9^{199}	Aspartame	Omega3	ENV/GBLV Homeopathic (Z)
12.9^{999}	Toxic Gold	Vitamin E	Bio-3-BG (BR)

Frequency Range >12.9^{1000} and <12.9^{2000}

Frequency	Toxin	Deficiency	Supplement/Company*
12.9^{1003}	Glyphosate	Tissue Cell Salts	L-Lysine HCL (BR)
12.9^{1004}	Mercury/ Aluminum Compound	Trace Mineral	GB Complete (Z)
12.9^{1899}	Sodium Lauryl Sulfate	Potassium	MSM Plus (Z)
12.9^{1999}	Aflatoxins	Vitamin C	ENV/GBLV Homeopathic (Z)

Continued next page

Toxin Chart (by Frequency), continued

\multicolumn{4}{c}{Frequency Range >12.9^{2000} and <12.9^{3000}}
Frequency	Toxin	Deficiency	Supplement/Company*
12.9^{2009}	MSG	Trace Mineral	ENV/GBLV Homeopathic (Z)
12.9^{2099}	Formaldehyde	Vitamin C	ENV/GBLV Homeopathic (Z)
12.9^{2199}	Parabens	Calcium	GSH Plus (BR)
12.9^{2599}	Nitrates	Mag/Cal/ Potassium receptors	Dysbiocide (BR)
12.9^{2799}	Insecticides	B Complex	GB Complete (Z) Beta Plus (BR)
$12.9^{2899.7}$	Pesticides	Magnesium	GB Complete (Z)
$12.9^{2899.9}$	Sulfates	Mag/Cal/ Potassium receptors	Bio-6-Plus (BR) or MSM Plus (Z)

CONTACT INFORMATION

For More Information:

- Appointment (tele-visit or in office): Call Health and Wellness of Carmel 317-663-7123, #1

- Email Questions for Dr. Weber: drjerrywebernd@gmail.com

- Videos and other information: www.drjerrywebernd.com and/or hwofc.com

- Facebook: Dr. Jerry Weber and/or Health and Wellness of Carmel

- YouTube: Dr Jerry Weber

For information on muscle testing classes or the online Certified Natural Health Practitioner program email request to drjerrywebernd@gmail.com

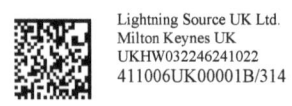